Clinical Research
for Health Professionals

D1515029

Clinical Research for Health Professionals

A User-Friendly Guide

Mitchell Batavia, Ph.D., P.T.

Assistant Professor of Physical Therapy, Department of Physical Therapy, School of Education, New York University, New York

BUTTERWORTH
HEINEMANN

Boston   Oxford   Auckland   Johannesburg   Melbourne   New Delhi

Copyright © 2001 by Butterworth–Heinemann

 A member of the Reed Elsevier group

All rights reserved.

No part of this publication may be reproduced, stored in a retrieval system, or transmitted in any form or by any means, electronic, mechanical, photocopying, recording, or otherwise, without the prior written permission of the publisher.

Every effort has been made to ensure that the drug dosage schedules within this text are accurate and conform to standards accepted at time of publication. However, as treatment recommendations vary in the light of continuing research and clinical experience, the reader is advised to verify drug dosage schedules herein with information found on product information sheets. This is especially true in cases of new or infrequently used drugs.

 Recognizing the importance of preserving what has been written, Butterworth–Heinemann prints its books on acid-free paper whenever possible.

 Butterworth–Heinemann supports the efforts of American Forests and the Global ReLeaf program in its campaign for the betterment of trees, forests, and our environment.

Library of Congress Cataloging-in-Publication Data

Batavia, Mitchell
    Clinical research for health professionals : a user-friendly guide / Mitchell Batavia.
       p. cm.
    Includes bibliographical references and index.
    ISBN 0-7506-7193-9 (alk. paper)
    1. Medicine—Research—Statistical methods—Handbooks, manuals, etc. 2. Clinical medicine—Research—Statistical methods—Handbooks, manuals, etc.
    [DNLM: 1. Research—methods. 2. Clinical Medicine—methods. 3. Statistics—methods. 4. Medical Errors. 5. Publishing. WB 25 B328c 2001]
    R853.S7 B37 2001
    610'.7'2—dc21

                                                                                              00-031219

British Library Cataloguing-in-Publication Data
A catalogue record for this book is available from the British Library.

The publisher offers special discounts on bulk orders of this book.
For information, please contact:

Manager of Special Sales
Butterworth-Heinemann
225 Wildwood Avenue
Woburn, MA 01801-2041
Tel: 800-366-2665
Fax: 781-904-2620

For information on all Butterworth–Heinemann publications available, contact our World Wide Web home page at: http://www.bh.com

10 9 8 7 6 5 4 3 2 1

Printed in the United States of America
The cover: Brown and orange earth colors were influenced by the artist, Amadeo Modigliani.

NB
25
3328c
2001

To my father, Gabriel, for encouraging a variety of interests in my life.
And, to my mother, Renée, for instilling the importance of education in my early years.

Contents

Preface

Clinical Research for Health Professionals is a conceptual approach to research education that entails a minimum of mathematics. It is a concise, mostly nontechnical manual that offers a fresh approach to understanding, appreciating, and conducting research in a nonthreatening way with metaphors, visual images, and entertaining examples. It is the kind of text I wish I had when I was in graduate school.

Although a plethora of research books exist, few if any of these books address major problems of conducting good research in a *nontechnical, visually oriented, user-friendly way*. Using metaphors, the reader is provided with the ultimate reasons why some research is lauded while other research is trashed.

Students often spend countless hours or years reading research textbooks several times before they become familiar with the jargon and acquainted with critical issues in conducting research. Eventually, they master the jargon, recite research dogma, and even perform death-defying statistical gymnastics without ever developing a visceral sense of what it means to do good research. As a result, students are often at a loss when attempting to evaluate their own study or deciding whether their patients will benefit from others' research.

Clinical Research for Health Professionals is ideal for undergraduate students having their first brush with research or for graduate students trying to fill gaps in their research education. The manual can serve as a foundation for planning projects and perhaps make the journey into the world of measurement more enjoyable, or at least much less painful.

The book can be used as a recommended text to supplement any introductory research course offered at the college level but *does not* serve as a replacement for a comprehensive research methods or statistics textbook.

Finally, the book can be useful to clinicians who desire guidelines for reading journal articles, applying results to patient care, taking the first steps toward reporting a case or establishing reliability in their clinics. The book also may provide clinicians with a nonthreatening window into the world of hypothesis testing. (Interestingly, clinicians test hypotheses in the clinic every time they evaluate the effect of a treatment on a patient. This kind of thinking process, which is emphasized more in research than clinical education, simply needs to be nurtured, developed, and formalized.)

Clinical Research for Health Professionals tackles the goal of understanding research much as a clinician would go about understanding a patient's problem: Before you can diagnose a medical problem, you need to understand anatomy, physiology, and pathology. This book may help you do the same for healthy and sick research reports.

The book is organized into five parts. Part I (Chapters 1 and 2) focuses on the unique purpose of research—to produce believable new knowledge using the scientific method. Chapter 1 discusses a metaphor, a boat, that may be useful in understanding how important it is for investigators to minimize mistakes in their methods so that their findings will be credible. Chapter 2 discusses five sources of acquiring knowledge: authority, trial and error, tradition, reasoning, and the scientific method. Of the five sources, the scientific method offers the most credible means of acquiring new knowledge.

Part II (Chapters 3 through 14) covers the structure and function of the research process. Learning the structure and function of research is somewhat analogous to learning the anatomy and physiology of the human body before understanding the pathology. Topics include understanding questions and how to conduct a literature search, hypotheses, theory, design, sampling, measurement, statistical analysis, and hypothesis testing.

Part II also includes two unique features not typically found in many research books. In Chapters 10 through 12, important statistical concepts are illustrated with computer exercises. The reader can enter data into a statistical spreadsheet and observe how different data affect the outcome of an analysis. In Chapter 13, examples of how to link questions, designs, and statistical analyses are provided. Making the connection between these research components seems to be an area in which graduate students have some difficulty.

Part III (Chapters 15 through 20) covers the different kinds of mistakes that can be committed in research and suggests ways to "vaccinate" or protect a study from these destructive forces. The concepts of internal and external validity are emphasized and potential mistakes are highlighted in six practical categories: investigators, treatments, subjects, measurements, measurements over time, and math.

In Part IV, Chapter 21 discusses how to critique a research report. In Chapter 22, a previously published, peer-reviewed research article is included to highlight where to locate different parts of a report.

Finally, in Part V, separate chapters are dedicated to the clinician and the graduate student. Chapter 23, for clinicians, suggests how to start a journal club, how to establish reliability of measurement in the clinic, and how to write and present case reports. Computer exercises for conducting intrarater and interrater reliability analyses are reviewed. I believe clinicians will gain a better understanding of reliability issues by analyzing some data, that is, learn by doing. Such experiences may help to forge the wide gap between clinician and researcher, to foster collaboration, and ultimately lead clinicians to practice and think more scientifically, to become clinician–researchers. Chapter 24, for graduate students, reviews desirable attributes of a graduate student and ways to excel in or at least survive the graduate experience. In Chapter 25, I present my vision of a fruitful collaboration between clinicians and researchers.

Appendix A lists recommended books and resources for conducting Internet searches, for research designs, and for statistical analysis. Appendix B is a fairly exhaustive list that defines the many kinds of biases (mistakes) that can be committed in research. The list is an appendix from a previously published journal article authored by David L. Sackett. Such a list will certainly give the reader a scope of the problems facing the researcher in conducting credible work.

Clinical Research for Health Professionals is aimed to pique the reader's interest in clinical research. If this material, even in some small way, eases the pain of graduate school education or leads to productive collaboration between researchers and clinicians, then my mission is accomplished.

M. B.

Acknowledgments

I thank the publisher, Butterworth–Heinemann; my medical editors, Mary Drabot, Leslie Kramer, and Cheri Dellelo; and Jodie Allen, Production Editor, for helping this work come to fruition.

I thank reviewers for their comments and generous donation of time for one or more chapters: Charles Sprague, Carl Mason, and the reviewers from Butterworth-Heinemann. Special thanks to Dr. Rosamond Gianutsos for her very helpful review of the statistics chapters, insights into Jacob Cohen's writings, and her suggestion of adding computer statistical exercises to the text. I thank Dr. John G. Gianutsos, Director of Research, Department of Rehabilitation, NYU School of Medicine, for serving as my mentor over the years and guiding me in some of my classic literature; and to Dr. Sharon L. Weinberg for the use of her metaphor on statistical power—the dimmer.

I thank the administration of the NYU School of Education for their support in funding a drawing course, which assisted me in completing illustrations for the book. I thank my students at NYU who through their feedback helped me to identify and include meaningful content areas in the book. I also acknowledge past support from the Department of Education National Institute of Disability and Rehabilitation Research grant for physical therapy clinical research; Robert Salant post-doctoral fellowship; and Dr. Wen Ling, chairperson of the Department of Physical Therapy, School of Education, NYU, for her support and guidance.

Although the aforementioned individuals and many others who mentored me during my research training have either directly or indirectly influenced my writing, I alone take full responsibility for any deficiencies.

Part I
How to Use This Book and Overview

Clinical Research for Health Professionals tackles the goal of understanding research much as a clinician would go about understanding a patient's problem. Before you can diagnose a medical problem, you need to be well versed in anatomy, physiology, and pathology. This book may help you do the same for healthy and sick research reports.

The book is organized into five parts. If you are completely new to research, read Parts I and II first. The chapters end with sections called "Things to Do," which encourages activities that help consolidate learning. Graduate students trying to fill in missing pieces in their education should feel free to skip around as needed.

Part I focuses on the purpose of research—to acquire believable new knowledge using the scientific method. A boat metaphor is provided to underscore the importance of reducing errors in a study so that the findings remain credible.

Part II, structure and function, discusses fundamental concepts in research needed to critique a report in journal club or in the planning of a research project. Chapter 4 discusses how to review the literature and conduct searches over the Internet. A recommended list of books and resources for conducting searches also is included in Appendix A. Chapters 10 through 12 covers statistical concepts by having you actually enter data into a statistical spreadsheet (if available) to observe the outcome of analyses. If you do not have access to a statistical software package, you can still benefit from the material.

Part III, pathology, discusses the kinds of mistakes that can be committed in research and suggests particular ways to "vaccinate" or protect your study from these destructive forces. These chapters may be particularly useful for graduate students planning a study or clinicians who are critiquing the strengths and weaknesses of a report. Part III also includes a section on internal and external validity, which is crucial when evaluating the quality of a research report.

Part IV, examination, discusses in detail how to critique a research report. In Chapter 22, a previously published, peer-reviewed article is included to highlight the location of different parts of a research report.

In Part V, separate chapters are dedicated to clinicians and graduate students. For clinicians, starting a journal club, establishing reliability in the clinic, and writing and presenting case reports are discussed. For graduate students who need to complete a thesis or dissertation, tips on surviving and perhaps maximizing their educational experience are discussed.

This book may help students make the journey through graduate school more enjoyable, make clinicians better consumers of the literature, and perhaps encourage clinicians to take the first steps toward writing case reports. Ultimately, an author seeks a healthy research collaboration between clinicians and academics so that in the end the patient benefits.

1

The Boat Metaphor

THE BIG PICTURE: MAKING A STUDY BELIEVABLE

Ultimately it comes down to either believing or not believing the findings of a study. Mistakes made during a study compromise the validity (soundness) of the conclusions and lead to disbelief in the report. A boat metaphor is used in this chapter to help you understand the overall challenge of the researcher—to acquire new knowledge in a believable way.

THE BOAT METAPHOR

Imagine you are out rowing and have found an extremely interesting object on a remote island. You place the object on the deck of your boat, head for home, and continue to study the object along the way. To get home, however, you need to navigate treacherous waters filled with icebergs (Figure 1-1).

Each of the icebergs represents a kind of mistake that you can make in your efforts to study the object. These potential mistakes are numerous and can include problems with measuring (reliability), math (statistics), sampling, conducting studies over time, or a preconceived notion of the object (your bias). The predicament you face is arriving home (finishing the study) without bumping into any of the icebergs along the way (mistakes in research). Each time you crash into an iceberg, you make a hole in your boat. Water leaks in and submerges your precious object, making it more difficult to see and study. The more icebergs you bump into, the more water leaks into the boat and the less capable you are to study the object. When enough water leaks in (lots of mistakes), the boat sinks. Your study *does not float anymore*. At this point, even if you reach some conclusions about the object, no one would believe your findings because you have made too many mistakes (bumped into too many icebergs) along the way.

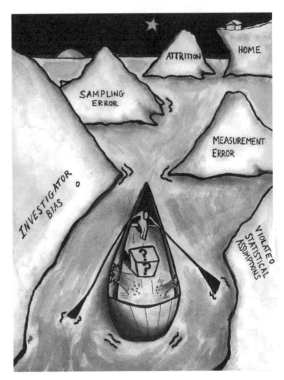

Figure 1-1. The boat metaphor. The journey in research can be treacherous with many potential icebergs (mistakes) that can sink your boat (study) along the way.

LOCATING MISTAKES

Mistakes in research can *sink your boat*, rendering your study less believable. Most of these mistakes can be found in the methods and results sections of journal articles.

GOAL OF THE RESEARCHER

The goal of the researcher is to conduct a study and report results that are believable (valid) by avoiding or minimizing mistakes (metaphorical icebergs) that can undermine the study. The purpose of this book is to point out when these mistakes are likely to occur and suggest effective vaccinations (protection) to maintain the health of your study.

THINGS TO DO

Create your own metaphor concerning mistakes that can threaten the believability of a study. If the boat metaphor does not work for you, invent your own. For example, you can draw parallels between the research process and Homer's *Odyssey*. In this case, the goal of the investigator is to avoid encounters with the Cyclopes and the Sirens (mistakes in research) that may ultimately destroy you and your crew (the credibility of the study) or prevent you from returning home.

2

Why Research?

Ultimately all knowledge originates from five sources: (1) tradition, (2) authority, (3) trial and error, (4) reasoning, and (5) scientific method.[1] This is true whether you search for answers in textbooks, dictionaries, encyclopedias, on the Internet, or from professors. The scientific method incorporates elements of the other four methods of acquiring knowledge. Of the five sources, the scientific method offers the most credible knowledge base because it uses objective, observable, and probabilistic means to acquire new knowledge.

FIVE SOURCES OF KNOWLEDGE

TRADITION

One way to gain knowledge is to do what, by tradition, has been done before. Perhaps tradition transmits knowledge so that knowledge does not have to be reinvented for each new generation. To that end, tradition has served as a to guide to clinical practice in rehabilitation.[1] Tradition is not always a bad way to gain knowledge. Acupuncture, for example, has been developed and practiced by the Chinese for more than 2000 years. It has been shown effective in pain management as evident by reports of using acupuncture during operations performed without anesthetics.[2]

On the other hand, tradition can have limitations. Traditional practices may be based on superstition or misguided theory, such as bloodletting and trephination. Bloodletting, an ineffective tradition of bleeding patients, has origins in ancient Greece. It was believed to help correct imbalances in the humors that circulated in the blood.[3] Surprisingly, this practice actually continued well into the middle of the 19th century.

Another example of tradition gone wrong is trephination, the ancient medical practice of carving a 2.5 to 5 cm

hole in the skull of a person suffering from insanity or headaches. Trephination was believed to secure a cure by driving out evil spirits, although I'm not quite sure how carving into the skull would relieve a headache.[4] Finally, the ancients practiced a form of birth control that entailed having the woman jump backward seven times immediately after coitus. I would not try this at home.[4]

In summary, although tradition can serve to transmit useful knowledge from past to future generations, it may also propagate useless and potentially harmful practices if left unchallenged.

AUTHORITY

Authority is a second way to gain knowledge. Because authoritarian figures may manipulate knowledge to their personal advantage, one should exercise caution when believing persons in power. In the 1600s, the Roman Catholic Church (the authority) insisted that Galileo renounce his idea that the Earth revolved around the Sun because this concept was not consistent with church teaching.[5] In Nazi Germany, the authority (the Nazis) deemed Albert Einstein and his ideas unacceptable and decided to remove him from his university post.[6,7] In the 1920s, John Scopes was put on trial (the Tennessee monkey trial) for teaching evolution to students.[6]

Powerful figures can have a lasting influence in our understanding and practice of medicine. For example, Galen (c.130–c.200), a Greek physician and authority on medicine in ancient Rome, taught that the nervous system was glandular (not electrical) in nature[3] and that the blood ebbed and flowed rather than circulated through the body.[4,6] Such misconceptions persisted for hundreds of years. In the 19th century, the medical community was unduly influenced by Hilton's book on the importance of rest in the management of pain after accidents.[8,9] Using anecdotes, Hilton recommended rest for a wide range of medical problems, including injuries attributed to falls and concussions. Remarkably, the book was in print for almost 100 years, the latest edition being published in the 1950s. We now know that immobilization can lead to many unnecessary complications, including connective tissue shortening.[10]

On the other hand, getting advice from an authority sometimes is a good idea if the information comes from a good source. If you were in the Land of Oz and needed information on how to get home, you would go no farther than the authority, the Wizard. A doctoral student who has difficulty finishing a dissertation may seek the advice from a committee member, probably an expert. If you are developing a new questionnaire, it is not uncommon to ask a panel of experts (authorities) for their opinions on the merits of the new test (content validity).[1] Finally, research reports must include citations to trace and credit knowledge derived from authoritative sources.

In summary, although authorities may be the source of useful information, the potential for abuse, as evident from the past, suggests some caution in accepting opinion from these individuals at face value in the future.

TRIAL AND ERROR

Trial and error is another means of acquiring knowledge, although it may take the investigator a long time before he or she arrives at the truth using this approach. In other words, you may have to commit many errors before one of your trials ends in success. Infants use trial and error to acquire knowledge about rolling, sitting, and walking during their development.[11] Luther Burbank, a 19th century plant breeder, had great success improving crops and producing new varieties of fruits using a hit-and-miss method of pollination.[12] In contrast, Gregor Mendel used planned, scientific methods to investigate the inherited characteristic of peas.[13] Finally, a pilot study, which can be viewed as a dress rehearsal for a study, involves trial and error to identify problems that may arise in an actual experiment.

REASONING

Reasoning (the use of logic) is another source of knowledge. The scientific method entails both deductive and inductive reasoning during research. In the following example, the central pattern generator (neural circuits in the spinal cord believed to organize the pattern of locomotion) is used to illustrate deductive and inductive reasoning.

Deductive Reasoning

Given a general principle (a theory), you predict future observations (the particulars).[1,14] For example, if you believe that the neural control for locomotion is located in the spinal cord of all mammals (central pattern generator theory) and you see a new mammal, you may claim that

the locomotor mechanism of this new mammal also is located at the spinal cord level.[15]

Deductive reasoning often is used in the *introductory portion* of a research report when investigators want to test a general principle and claim (hypothesize) that on the basis of this general principle, one would expect certain observations or relationships to be found in the study. Consider the following example in an introduction section of a hypothetical report: "It is generally believed that the mechanism for locomotion resides in the spinal cord of animals. Thus, in this newly discovered species of mammal, I expect their locomotor mechanism to also be located in the spinal cord."

If the general principle is incorrect, such as that health requires a balance of humors in the blood and balance is accomplished through bloodletting, then predictions will not be accurate, such as "if I bleed him, he will recover."[6]

Inductive Reasoning

Given enough data (the particulars), you develop a general principle (a theory).[1,14] For example, if you find, after extensive sampling, that mammals of all kinds from all over the world have spinal level activity attributed to locomotion, you can make a generalization that all mammals rely on a spinal cord mechanism for walking (central pattern generator theory).[15]

Inductive reasoning often is used in the *discussion portion* of a research report because investigators are attempting to make sense of their data and to develop a general principle or theory. Consider the following example in the discussion section of a hypothetical report: "Data from 15 different species of spinal mammal preparations suggest that the basic wiring for locomotion resides in the spinal cord, thus supporting the notion of a central pattern generator."

Keep in mind that if the data are incorrect (if some of your subjects were not mammals but actually marine animals such as sponges), your general principle may be too inclusive (sponges cannot possibly rely on a locomotor mechanism that originates in the spine because they are spineless).

THE SCIENTIFIC METHOD

The scientific method is a credible means of acquiring new knowledge because it relies on objective observations. With this method, probability (the likelihood that an event will occur) is used to determine whether a phenomenon (potential knowledge) can be generalized or is simply due to chance. Other knowledge sources tend to be less objective (authority and traditions often are not challenged), to lack careful planning (trial and error can be haphazard), or lack data (reasoning is not confirmed with actual data).

Shortcomings of the Scientific Method

The scientific method has shortcomings. First, science cannot answer all questions in life. For example, philosophical questions such as: Is there a creator? What is the purpose of life? or Is there a life after death? cannot be answered with the scientific method.[1] It is not that these questions are unimportant. It is just that there is no way to objectively observe and measure phenomena about such questions. Even if you have had a subjective observation, such as a near-death experience, you still would be hard pressed to measure or persuade others of your observation in an objective way.[16]

Second, findings from a research study are only as good as the quality of the work that went into the study. If the investigator was biased, the study poorly conceived, or other mistakes were committed (humans can do that), findings will be meaningless, misleading, or unbelievable.

Incorporating Other Sources of Knowledge

Although the scientific method is the most credible source of new knowledge, other sources are incorporated. For example, logic is used deductively to test a hypothesis at the beginning of a study and is used inductively to formulate theory at the end of the experiment. Persons with authority are cited in the literature review, and trial and error methods may be used during the early planning stages of the experiment (pilot study). Even tradition (e.g., publications, poster presentations) serves as a means of communicating new knowledge produced in a study.

Which Knowledge Source Came First? The lines that differentiate the origins of knowledge may not always be clear. Imagine you are summoned to care for a king's painful shoulder and you accidentally relocate this joint back into its socket through trial and error. You later reason that the joint was most stable when manipulated into that particular position (a feat of logic). The king is impressed with your technique and commands it as the official first aid of the kingdom (authority has spoken). The technique continues to be used for hundreds of years (tradition transmits). Finally, one day someone tests the technique for efficacy by using a comparison group (objective science is born). Although this scenario may appear attractive to some (blending all knowledge sources into a well-fitting package), the true history of knowledge should probably be left to the historians.

THINGS TO DO

1. Chart the strengths and weakness of (a) traditional, (b) authoritative, (c) trial and error, (d) reasoning, or (e) scientific sources of knowledge. Give an original example of each knowledge source.

2. Identify a treatment approach (e.g., exercise approach, medication, surgery) in your field. Then identify the source of knowledge used to develop that particular approach (tradition, authority, trial and error, reasoning, scientific method).

3. Identify three clinical problems (e.g., pressure ulcer, spasticity, depression) and proposed solutions in your field. Are the effects of these proposed solutions (a) observable and (b) measurable? That is, can they be addressed with the scientific method?

REFERENCES

1. Portney LG, Watkins MP. *Foundations of Clinical Research: Applications to Practice.* Upper Saddle River, N.J.: Prentice Hall; 2000.
2. Payton OD. *Research: The Validation of Clinical Practice.* Philadelphia: FA Davis; 1979.
3. McGrew RE. *Encyclopedia of Medical History.* New York: McGraw-Hill; 1985.
4. *New Encyclopedia Britannica.* 15th ed., s.v. "medicine," p. 775.
5. *Random House Webster's Dictionary of Scientists.* New York: Random House; 1997.
6. Beveridge WIB. *The Art of Scientific Investigation.* 3rd ed. New York: Vintage Books; 1957.
7. Muir H. *Larousse Dictionary of Scientists.* Edinburgh: Larousse; 1994.
8. Hilton J. *On the Influence of Mechanical and Physiological Rest in the Treatment of Accidents and Surgical Diseases, and the Diagnostic Value of Pain.* London: Bell & Daldy, 1950.
9. Cyriax J. *Diagnosis of Soft Tissue Lesions.* 7th ed. London: Baillieres Tindall; 1979. *Textbook of Orthopaedic Medicine.* Vol 1.
10. Akeson WH, Amiel D, Woo SLY. Immobility effects on synovial joints: the pathomechanics of joint contractures. *Biorheology.* 1980;17:95–110.
11. Feldenkrais M. *Body and Mature Behavior: A Study of Anxiety, Sex, Gravitation, and Learning.* New York: International University Press; 1949.
12. Howard WL. *Luther Burbank: a victim of hero worship. Chronica Botanica.* 1945;9:358.
13. Hart MH. *The 100: A Ranking of the Most Influential Persons in History.* Secaucus, NJ: Citadel Press; 1987.
14. Light RJ, Singer JD, Willett JB. *By Design: Planning Research on Higher Education.* Cambridge, Mass: Harvard University Press, 1990.
15. Peterson I. *The Jungles of Randomness: A Mathematical Safari.* New York: John Wiley & Sons; 1998.
16. Giere RN. *Understanding Scientific Reasoning.* 4th ed. Fort Worth, Tex: Harcourt Brace College; 1997.

Part II
Anatomy and Physiology: Understanding Research Concepts

Part II covers fundamental concepts in research. If you are new to research, do not skip these chapters. Statistical concepts are demonstrated with computer exercises. Issues such as questions, designs, and analyses are treated in separate chapters and are addressed together in Chapter 13.

3

Anatomy: Understanding the Research Process

It is important to know the anatomy of the research process just as a surgeon needs to know anatomy of the human body before he or she starts cutting. That way, if something goes wrong during a study, you can locate the problem or at least prevent it from occurring the next time.

PHASES OF A RESEARCH STUDY

The research process is typically described as comprising five main phases. These phases include (1) developing a question, (2) developing a method to answer the question, (3) collecting data, (4) analyzing, interpreting, and reflecting on the data, and (5) sharing the information.[1,2] These phases can be divided into more detailed stages.

ALTERNATIVE WAYS OF SEEING RESEARCH

Whereas the five phases of research are fine, this description seems to lack the spirit of the research process. In other words, it fails to convey the anticipation, excitement, and surprise investigators often experience when doing research. I therefore suggest alternative ways of appreciating the research process that incorporates the notion of *fun* (you read that correctly *fun*).

First, it helps to simplify the research process into only three major phases. I use the humanities (film and music) as metaphors to better appreciate the dynamic phases of research. My hope is that you will be able to appreciate the links between science and the humanities and to realize that there are common threads to solving problems for life's many human endeavors.[3,4]

THREE PHASES OF RESEARCH

It may be helpful to describe the three phases of research by comparing them with the introduction,

methods, and results and discussion sections of a research report (Figure 3-1).

The Beginning Phase: The Introduction of a Report

The beginning phase of research (the introduction of a report) includes the question, hypothesis, and theory. The question drives the entire study. It is the problem you want to solve. The hypothesis is your tentative answer to the problem. It is the prediction that provides suspense and sustains your interest throughout the study. The theory is the investigator's rationale for the hypothesis or prediction (e.g., you can get to the East by sailing west because the earth is round). According to the boat metaphor, the beginning phase of research includes looking at the rare object, formulating an idea about what it is, and stating a hypothesis that allows you to test your idea.

The Middle Phase: The Methods Section of a Report

The middle phase of research (methods section of a research report) involves answering the question through observation or experimentation. This phase includes the design (blueprint or plan), instrumentation, and the procedures used to collect data (your evidence). In the boat

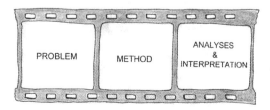

Figure 3-1. The research process can be likened to a film or book. Each has a beginning (the problem), a middle (method), and an end (analysis and interpretation).

metaphor, you plot out a safe course to your home destination so that you can analyze your object.

The Final Phase: The Results, Discussion, Conclusion Sections of a Report

The final phase of research (results, discussion, and conclusion sections) involves analyzing the data and interpreting the data (making sense of them) so that the question can finally be answered. In the boat metaphor, you determine whether your evidence matches your suspicion of what you believed the object to be. On the basis of your new finding and the repeated confirmations of others, this new knowledge may eventually find its way into journals, books, and encyclopedias.

USING FILMS AND BOOKS TO UNDERSTAND THE RESEARCH PROCESS

You can usually also divide a film or book into three parts—a beginning, a middle, and an end.[5]

The Beginning of the Story: The Problem or Situation

The beginning of the story establishes the problem or situation. The situation may be two people from opposite sides of the track who fall in love (Romeo and Juliet);[6] an underdog Italian club boxer with a shot at the world champion heavyweight title (Rocky);[7] or a cafe owner in Morocco during World War II who wants to leave the country (Casablanca).[7] The important point is that the situation creates tension and catches the interest of the audience.

In a similar way, research begins with a situation (a problem) that has to be solved. The researcher develops a question to address the problem. The problem may be to determine which of two popular therapeutic interventions is more effective or whether an association exists between the water we drink and some forms of cancer. Or perhaps the problem is to determine which of two popular theories (gate theory or endorphin theory) best explains the effects of acupuncture. If the research problem is important enough, it will capture the interest of both the researcher and the reader.

The Middle of the Story: The Conflict

The middle of a story is characterized by a building, intensification, and increasing conflict in the situation. In *Romeo and Juliet,* bad blood between the two families prevents the lovers from making a life together. In the film *Rocky,* the underdog fighter trains against seemingly unbeatable odds and loses the initial rounds of the boxing match. In *Casablanca,* Rick's desire for his old lover places him in conflict with his patriotism.

Similarly, as a research project develops, interest increases when conflict exists. The investigator is now actively planning a solution to the problem, and the suspense of anticipating the outcome helps to sustain the

interest of the investigator through the rest of the study. For example, recruitment flyers are being posted, newspapers are advertising the study, potential subjects are inquiring about the study, and you begin data collection with your first subjects.

The End of the Story: Resolution of the Problem

The end of a story is characterized by the resolution of the conflict. In *Romeo and Juliet,* the two lovers cannot have a life together so they choose death. In *Rocky,* the underdog overcomes seemingly unbeatable odds, wins the title, and becomes the heavyweight boxing champion of the world. In Casablanca, Rick's patriotism wins out over his self-interest and the desire for his old lover.

In research, the problem is resolved during the analysis phase of the study when it is finally determined which intervention is better, whether an association truly exists, or whether one or another theory provides the best explanation of reality.

USING MUSIC TO UNDERSTAND THE RESEARCH PROCESS

If you are more music than film buff, you may be able to draw on music to gain insight into the dynamics of the research process.[8,9] The opening movement of a sonata, for example, often uses contrasting themes or musical ideas to engage the interest of the audience. The contrasting themes provide tension in the music that ultimately is resolved, much as a problem addressed in a study is resolved.

For a taste of contrasting ideas or themes in music, put on a lab coat, close your eyes, and listen to the first movement of either Beethoven's Fifth Symphony or Mozart's *Eine kleine Nachtmusik.* Draw yourself into the first theme, then the opposing lighter theme. Notice how the two themes interweave a story and develop into a climactic showdown in which one idea ultimately triumphs over the other, ending in an unambiguous outcome.

The Sonata

The Exposition. The exposition, the opening section of a sonata consists of two opposing or contrasting themes in two different keys. The themes, in a sense, are exposing or revealing themselves. The first theme is considered masculine and the contrasting theme feminine or idyllic. These two themes can be clearly identified in Beethoven's Fifth Symphony. In a similar way, research begins with a question. The question may involve two contrasting ideas or theories that are attempts to explain reality. The goal of the investigator is to determine which of the ideas or theories best explains reality.

The Development. In the development, the second section of a sonata, tension between the two contrasting themes gradually builds in excitement until it reaches a dramatic, maximum intensity. In the research process, one can envision excitement and anticipation building as the planning phase of the study reaches its conclusion, and the two conflicting theories are finally ready to be put to the test. That is, the investigator is preparing to see which theory is more valid by collecting and analyzing evidence derived from an experiment.

The Recapitulation.   In the recapitulation, the final section of the movement, tension abates as the two opposing themes reconcile with a *wealth of new meaning*. During the analysis phase of research, the investigator hopes to reach a decision (resolution) regarding which of two theories is most useful in explaining reality.

RESEARCH DOES NOT END

Unlike the end of a movie or the final movement in a sonata, the research process rarely ends. Findings from studies often lead to new questions and additional studies that continue to provide us with a richer, deeper understanding of our world.

COMMON MISTAKES IN THINKING ABOUT RESEARCH

MY STUDY WILL CHANGE THE WORLD

A common mistake is thinking that research begins and ends with one study and that your study will be the definitive one that will change the world. The cold reality is that your study is simply one building block in a series of studies that may *gradually* provide a new way to view a phenomenon.[10]

RESEARCH IS A SEQUENCE OF STEPS

Another mistake is thinking of research as a series of steps completed much as someone completes a paint-by-number art project. Although an experiment is methodical, an investigator often works simultaneously on many portions of a study (e.g., the literature review, developing instrumentation, planning subject recruitment) much as an artist works different portions of a canvas at the same time until the painting matures and emerges as a finished work. Thus, much of research can be an exciting, dynamic process of problem solving for those who approach it in this manner.

THINGS TO DO

1. Choose a research report. (a) Identify the introduction, methods, and results, discussion, and conclusion sections of the research article. (b) List the issues discussed in each section of the report. (c) List activities in which the investigator may have engaged in the beginning, middle, and final portions of the research.
2. Choose a sonata or first movement of a symphony *that you enjoy*. (a) Play the musical piece and try to identify the three sections: the exposition, development, and recapitulation. (b) Identify the two conflicting themes in the exposition. (c) Notice the resolution of tension in the recapitulation. (d) See whether you can draw an analogy between the tension in music with opposing views of a problem identified in the introduction section of the research report chosen for question 1.
3. Recall a film, novel, or short story. (a) Identify the beginning, middle, and end of the story. (b) Identify the problem that had to be resolved in the beginning of the story. (c) Notice how the problem resolved itself toward the end of the story. (d) Draw an analogy between the problem in the story and the problem identified in the research report chosen for question 1.

REFERENCES

1. Portney LG, Watkins MP. *Foundations of Clinical Research: Applications to Practice.* Upper Saddle River, N.J.: Prentice Hall; 2000.
2. Payton OD. *Research: The Validation of Clinical Practice.* Philadelphia: FA Davis; 1979.
3. Luft R, Löw H. Excellence and creativity in science. *Clin Res.* 1980;28:329–337.
4. Fischer EP. Art and science. *Nature.* 1997;390:330.
5. Hauge M. *Writing Screenplays That Sell.* New York: HarperCollins; 1991.
6. Boyle C, ed. *Shakespeare A to Z: The Essential Reference to His Plays, His Poems, His Life, and Times, and More.* New York: Facts on File; 1990.
7. Ebert R. *Roger Ebert's Video Companion 1998.* Kansas City, Mo: Andrews McMeel Universal; 1997.
8. Machlis J. *The Enjoyment of Music: An Introduction to Perceptive Listening.* 5th ed. New York: WW Norton; 1984.
9. Rosen C. *Sonata Forms.* New York: WW Norton; 1980.
10. Harre, R. *Great Scientific Experiments: 20 Experiments that Changed Our View of the World.* Oxford, England: Phaidon; 1981.

4

Questions

The first step in conducting research is to identify a question. Identifying a good question is one of the most difficult tasks in doing research and requires patience and perseverance. One usually starts with a general problem area and later whittles it down to a tiny question that can be answered in one study.

QUESTIONS IN BASIC AND APPLIED RESEARCH

There are two types of research—basic and applied. Basic research involves pursuing a question for the sake of intellectual curiosity, perhaps to develop a theory or simply study a phenomenon to learn more about it. The investigator is not overly concerned whether the findings will help society. Although the findings may contribute to important problems in the future, this is not necessarily what motivates the investigator. Applied research, one the other hand, involves answering questions to solve problems in society.[1] A common thread is that in both types of research, investigators are trying to acquire new knowledge by answering a question. In this clinically oriented book, questions are of a practical, clinical nature, and theory (see Chapter 6) will be used as a requisite to achieving better understanding of the problem.

STEP ONE: IDENTIFY A GENERAL PROBLEM

Problems in life motivate us to ask questions (i.e., necessity is the mother of invention). There are three good places to identify a general problem: (1) your patients, (2) lectures and articles, and (3) existing theory. Let's use the example of pressure ulcers as a general problem.[1,2]

YOUR PATIENTS

It is possible that you have become interested in the general problem of pressure ulcers because you have noticed that your patient's skin breaks down when he or she lies on a foam mattress, and the situation has upset you, not to mention the patient.[3]

LECTURES AND ARTICLES

You read an article in your journal that piques your interest. The investigator has found that patients with spinal cord injuries who used water mattresses (water beds) tended to have a low occurrence of pressure ulcers.

THEORY: EXISTING EXPLANATIONS FOR A PROBLEM

You may apply a theory (explanation) to your patient's problem. For example, Pascal's law predicts that pressure around a body part at a given height is equally distributed if surrounded by a fluid medium such as water. Because Pascal's law applies to water and perhaps to water beds, this can be an excellent way of developing a question. You may reason that because pressure ulcers may be caused in part by excess or unequal distribution of pressure over the skin and that because Pascal's law predicts equal distribution of water pressure around body parts, use of a water bed may reduce the frequency of pressure ulcers. Thus by looking at your patients, the literature, and existing theories, you have begun to identify a general problem area and can begin to refine the problem into a specific question.

IDENTIFYING OUTSTANDING PROBLEMS

Kahn[4] offers the following suggestions for identifying outstanding problems for research:

1. Imagine the most intriguing outcome of your study before you embark on it. If those results are not worth following up, abort that line of research.
2. If few colleagues believe your study is interesting, any favorable outcomes from the study probably will not

be viewed as remarkable or important in the research community.

3. Expose yourself to disciplines outside your area of specialization because you may gain a new perspective on a problem (theory, method, instrumentation) that can direct your future work. Too much familiarity with your own subject area may thwart efforts to think in different, more creative ways.

4. Be prepared to retool (go back to class) or collaborate with others to study new phenomena in depth. Retooling may mean updating your knowledge in motor learning, undergoing training with a new instrument, taking a refresher course in multivariate statistics, or learning a new programming language. Unfortunately, a common pattern among graduate students is simply to drop a variable they believe is beyond their ken.

CONDUCTING A LITERATURE SEARCH

A literature search is critical for developing your question, determining whether your question has already been answered, and staying current in your field. This section describes where to search for information using electronic (Internet, CD-ROM) and printed resources. Many of these resources can be accessed at medical, university, and large public libraries and through the Internet. Nine major search areas are as follows: (1) Internet searches, (2) journals, (3) health statistics, (4) government documents and technical reports, (5) dissertations, (6) papers presented at meetings, (7) people and organizations, (8) current events, and (9) textbooks. Useful sources of information are provided, but a more complete list of resources for conducting searches is provided in Appendix A. A search strategy is provided at the end of the section, as are considerations for evaluating information on the Internet.

Internet Searches

The Internet is a dynamic phenomenon. It grows rapidly every day. Learning basic search strategies is essential because Web addresses and methods of locating them are likely to change in the time it takes you to finish reading the words on this page. Just as we must rely on updated telephone directories to inform us of changes in telephone numbers and area codes, we should rely on electronic directory sources to locate old and new Web addresses on the Internet. Three general approaches to searching for information on the Internet involve the use of (1) subject directories, (2) search engines, and (3) meta-tools.[5,6] Each has its advantages.

Subject Directories. A *subject directory* is a good place to start if you are beginning a search and do not know the best key words to use. In a sense, you are browsing rather that searching. In subject directories, Web sites are organized by subject (or category). Searching is analogous to looking in the Yellow Pages under a general heading such as "Pharmacy." After you locate the subject, you can then explore individual drug stores, such as "Peter's Drugs," within the subject heading.[5]

Example of a Subject Directory

- Search: Yahoo
  (www.yahoo.com)

Search Engines. A *search engine*, which contains a huge database of Web sites through which to search, is a good approach if you know exactly what you are looking for, that is, you have an appropriate key word.[5] Using a search engine is analogous to searching for a specific name in a telephone book or index in the back of a book (e.g., Peter's Drugs). Just make sure you know the correct spelling of the key word.

Examples of Search Engines

- Search: AltaVista
  (www.altavista.com)
  Comment: Good for specific phrases
- Search: HotBot
  (www.hotbot.com)
  Comment: Offers many search options

Meta-Tools. A *meta-tool* can help if you want to cover a lot of ground in a general search for information.[5] A meta-tool looks for information simultaneously in many directories and search engines. This kind of search is analogous to looking in many phone books published by different companies. Some of the directories may have your information; others may not. When I became jaded because of failed attempts at using separate search engines and directories for information on "chickens that walk briefly following decapitation," someone in my department located this information with a meta-tool.

Examples of Meta-Tools

- Search: Dogpile
  (www.dogpile.com)
  Comment: A thorough and flexible meta-tool

Journals

Biomedical and Related Databases. Journal articles can be searched with print or electronic indexes. An advantage of electronic indexes (online; CD-ROM) is saving time. Many elements of a journal record (author, title, year, key word) can be searched simultaneously.[7] Once journal citations or abstracts are identified, the article can either be ordered online, requested as an interlibrary loan, or located in a medical library.

Of the electronic databases on the Internet, the National Library of Medicine (NLM) of the National Institutes of Health maintains more than 40 online databases, including MEDLINE, through a comprehensive, computerized system called MEDLARS (Medial Literature Analysis and Retrieval System).

The NLM offers two free online gateways to MED-LINE (PubMed and Internet Grateful Med), which may merge. PubMed's coverage of MEDLINE includes more than 4000 journal publications in the United States and 70 other countries (10 million citations and growing). It also provides links to online journals. Internet Grateful Med offers other databases in addition to MEDLINE, such as HealthStar, AIDSline, and Bioethicsline.[8]

Be aware that MEDLINE may not locate all research literature. For example, if you limit your search of randomized clinical trials to MEDLINE, you stand to miss about 50% of citations.[9] Search more than one database, not MEDLINE alone[7]; enter appropriate key words to search each database; and consider occasionally searching the journals themselves.

For additional information about PubMed and Internet Grateful Med, contact the NLM at 1 (888) FIND-NLM.[8]

- PubMed
  Search: PubMed
  (http://www.ncbi.nlm.nih.gov/PubMed/)
- Internet Grateful Med
  Search: Internet Grateful Med
  (http://igm.nlm.nih.gov/)

Databases in Internet Grateful Med

- MEDLINE
  Comment: For biomedical citations; primary online database for health; has the following print counterparts:
  - *Index Medicus.* Bethesda, Md: National Library of Medicine. Monthly. 1960–.
  - *International Nursing Index.* New York: American Journal of Nursing Company in cooperation with the National Library of Medicine. Quarterly. 1966–.
  - *Index to Dental Literature.* Chicago: American Dental Association and National Library of Medicine, Quarterly. 1962–.

- Histline
  Comment: For history of medicine citations
  AIDSline; AIDSdrugs, AIDStrials
  Comment: For AIDS citations
- Bioethicsline
  Comment: For ethics citations; also in print as *Bibliography of Bioethics*
- HealthSTAR
  Comment: For clinical and nonclinical citations
- STAR (Services, Technology, Administration, Research in health)
  Comment: In print as *Hospital and Health Administration Index*
- HSRPROJ
  Comment: For practice guidelines, health service, and technology citations

Other Databases

- CINAHL
  Comment: For allied health citations; printed as the *Cumulative Index to Nursing and Allied Health Literature.* Glendale, Calif: Glendale Adventist Medical Center. Bimonthly.[7] 1977–.
- PSYCHINFO
  Comment: For psychology citations; printed as *Psychological Abstracts.* Lancaster, Pa: American Psychological Association. Monthly. 1927–.[7]
- BIOSIS previews
  Comment: Printed as *Biological Abstracts.* Philadelphia: BioSciences Information Services. Biweekly. 1926–.[7]

Health Statistics

Statistics provide important information about the scope of a problem that can be cited in the introductory portion of a report (e.g., the number of falls that cause injuries).

Nongovernment and Government Agencies

- Search: Statistical Abstracts of the United States
  (http://www.census.gov/statab/www)
  Comment: Includes vital statistics for health, labor, and population[10]

International Sources

- Search: World Health Organization Statistical Information System (WHOSIS)
  (http://www.who.org/whosis)[10]

Federal Government Agencies

- Search: FEDSTATS
  (http://www.fedstats.gov)
  Click on A to Z; click on Health
  Comment: Locates U.S. statistics from more than 70 federal agencies[10]
- Search: U.S. Bureau of the Census
  (http://www.census.gov)[10]
  Comment: Statistics on aging, disability, population, demographics[10]
- Search: National Center for Health Statistics
  (http://www.cdc.gov/nchs)
- Search: OSHA home page
  (http://www.osha.gov)
  Comment: statistics on illness and injury rates[10]

Norms on Physical Measurements

Hall JG, Froster-Iskenius UG, Allanson JE. *Handbook of Normal Physical Measurements.* Oxford, England: Oxford University Press, 1991.
Comment: A printed source

U.S. Government Documents and Technical Reports

The U.S. government provides a wealth of often underused publications distributed by the Government Printing

Office (GPO) and are indexed in the Monthly Catalog of Publications. It is available over the Internet and in libraries.[7,8]

- Monthly Catalog of United States Government Publications. Washington, DC, U.S. Government Printing Office. Monthly; annual cumulative indexes. 1895–.
  Comment: The most comprehensive index of government publications
- Search: Monthly Catalog of Publications (MOCAT) Database list on GPO
  Access or click on Catalog of U.S. Government Publications (MOCAT)
  (http://www.access.gpo.gov/su_docs/db2.html)
  Comment: You can then conveniently search the nearest library to read the document.[8]

For technical reports, the U.S. government also has a National Technical Information Service that offers unclassified government-sponsored reports and research prepared by grantees, contractors, and federal agencies. The reports are indexed in Government Reports Announcements and Index.[7]

- Government Reports Announcements & Index. Springfield, Va: National Technical Information Service. April 4, 1975–.
- Search: National Technical Information Service (http://www.ntis.gov)
  Comment: Biweekly with annual cumulations

Dissertations

Dissertations, which are written by doctoral students in partial fulfillment of their degree requirements, offer scholarly research on a topic. Dissertations are reviewed for quality by university committees. Dissertations abstracts usually are available at university and large public libraries. Ask the librarian for Dissertations Abstracts International or a similar database. To purchase copies of U.S. dissertations contact

UMI Dissertation Services
300 North Zeeb Rd
Ann Arbor, MI 48106-1346
(800) 521-3042
(http://www.umi.com)

Papers Presented at Meetings, Reviews

Papers presented at meetings, whether published or unpublished, offer a current source of information.[7] Unpublished reports can serve as an important source of information (i.e., effect size) for use in meta-analyses.

Conference Papers Index. Bethesda, Md: Cambridge Scientific Abstracts. Monthly. 1973–.

Reviews provide an overview of a topic and can serve as both an introduction and an update of the knowledge base of a scientist.[7]

Bibliography of Medical Review. Bethesda, Md: National Library of Medicine. 1955–. It currently appears only as a separate section in Index Medicus.

People and Organizations

Sometimes the best means of acquiring information is "straight from the horse's mouth"—the expert. Sources from persons should be documented as an oral or written personal communication (see Appendix A for style manual resources).

- E-mail or write authors of journal reports (use correspondence information in journal articles).
- Write to authors through book publishers (I corresponded with Isaac Asimov this way).
- Use Web sites of authorities at universities and organizations on the Internet
- Go to professional conferences and meetings (refer to professional associations for announcements)
- Obtain information at continuing education courses (beware of speakers who pontificate but have little knowledge base ["the snake oil sellers"])
- Mail lists [5]

Mail lists are online discussion groups for specific topics (e.g., biomechanics). To participate, you must first subscribe to the list. Then any messages (questions) you post are forwarded to all subscribers, including experts, who may reply with a suggestion. To get off the list, you must unsubscribe. Follow instructions carefully for subscribing and unsubscribing.

Mail List Directory
- Search: Liszt
  (www.liszt.com)

To Contact Universities Around the World
- Search: Universities.com
  (www.universities.com)
  Comment: Lists 7500 (and growing) colleges and universities around the world[5]

To Contact Organizations and Government Offices
- Search: National Health Information Center
  (http://nhic-nt.health.org)
  Comment: Provides toll-free numbers
- Anders CE, Pearce LM, eds. Encyclopedia of Medical Organizations and Agencies. 9th ed. Detroit: Gaile Group; 2000.

Current Events

Searching for online news stories and press releases can keep you up to date with the latest information on a topic.

Press Releases
- Search: Newswise Search
  (http://www.newswise.com)
  Click on Med News; Search
  Comment: Provides press releases from research centers[11]

Health News Stories

- Search: CNN/Health
  Search CNN.com
  (http://www.cnn.com/HEALTH)
  Comment: Daily stories on health topics[11]

Textbooks and Libraries

Textbooks are sometimes the best place to begin a search. Libraries are the best resource for conducting searches in indexes when they cannot be located on the Internet. Librarians can be an excellent resource for locating and searching indexes.

Public Libraries

- Search: Library of Congress[11]
  (http://catalog.loc.gov)
  Click on Using the Library; click on Library of Congress Online Catalogs; select a search method
- Search: National Libraries
  (http://www.nlm.nih.gov/libraries/national.html)
- Search: Public Libraries with Internet Services
  Click on State; choose specific library
  (http://sjcpl.lib.in.us/homepage/PublicLibraries/
  PublicLibraryServers.html)
- Search: Eldredge Public Library[11]
  (http://www.capecod.net/epl)
  Click on Web Library Resources
  Click on Public Library Web sites in the United States

Medical Libraries

- Search: Medical research libraries by state
  (http://www.nlm.nih.gov/libraries/state.html)
  Comment: Access may be limited
- Search: Medical/Health Sciences Libraries on the Web[11]
  (http://www.arcade.uiowa.edu/hardin-www/hslibs.html)

University and Institutional Libraries

- Search: Library of Congress[11]
  (http://catalog.loc.gov)
  Click on Using the Library; click on Other Library Online Catalogs; click on Search other Catalogs

Book Publishers

- Search: AcqWeb's Directory of Publishers and Vendors
  (http://www.library.vanderbilt.edu/law/acqs/pubr.html)
  Comments: Contains directories for Web pages and e-mail addresses of book publishers

Search Strategy Example: Putting It All Together

One of many search strategies is presented for the graduate student and clinician. Imagine you want to search for information on pressure ulcers associated with use of wheelchairs by persons with quadriplegia. How would you start your search? Consider following these six steps:

1. Textbooks. Search medical textbooks and chapters in books to familiarize yourself with the literature and to identify key words (helpful search words). *Location:* medical, university, and large public libraries. If the book is 5 to 10 years old, contact the publisher to find out whether a new edition has been or is about to be published. In any case, look for relevant journal citations in the bibliography of the textbook.

2. Biomedical Journals. Include more than one biomedical database in your search. Search Medline, CINAH, HealthSTAR, STAR, and BIOSIS. Search for journal citations by key words (e.g., "pressure ulcer" AND quadriplegia AND wheelchair). *Location:* NLM Web site and libraries. The quotation marks are important because entering the words *pressure ulcer* without quotation marks, may result in a deluge of hits because both words, *pressure* and *ulcer,* will be searched independently. Refer to each database for suggestions on refining your search and selecting key words. If you get no results (called *hits*), broaden your search by reducing the search requirements by including alternative key words (e.g., "pressure sore," "spinal cord"); and ensuring that key words are spelled correctly.

If you get too many hits, narrow your search by limiting the search to the last few years, including an author's name in the search, or adding additional key words to the search. For example, include (AND "review article") in your search to read only reviews on the topic or (AND "clinical trial") if you wish to locate only articles involving therapeutic interventions.

3. Scholarly, Governmental, Organizational, and Health Statistical Sources. Search for dissertations and government publications. *Locations: Dissertation Abstracts* in libraries and MOCAT Web site, libraries. For additional leads, search and contact health organizations that champion a cause (e.g., a spinal cord injury association). For an overall sense of the prevalence of the problem (e.g., ulcers), search for health statistics. *Location:* FEDSTAT Web site; *Statistical Abstracts of the United States* Web site, and libraries.

4. Experts. Contact the author directly for clarification about article content using corresponding addresses and affiliations for research reports, through the publisher for books and chapters, through university directories, or through e-mail directories. If you are still stuck, consider posing your question to subscribers of a mail list with a special focus (e.g., paralysis). *Location:* Liszt.com. And don't forget the old-fashioned way of networking—talking—with colleagues at conferences. If you still have not located useful information, a knowledgeable research librarian can be of great assistance in generating a new search strategy.

5. Current Information. For recent news on the topic, check press releases (e.g., newswise.com) and news items (e.g., CNN.com).

6. Internet Searches.   For completeness, glean Web sites for additional information. As stated earlier, use a subject directory to browse, a search engine to search specific key words, or a meta-tool to cover a lot of ground. Because each directory or engine locates different Web sites, conducting a search in more than one subject directory or search engine is wise.[5]

Evaluating Internet Sources

To evaluate the quality of information on the Internet, consider the following:[5]

- The source. Is there bias? Government (.gov) and educational (.edu) affiliations, and well known organizations (.org), such as the American Heart Association are generally preferred over company (.com) sources, because companies may be trying to sell you something.
- E-mail contact information. Is the person an authority, and can he or she be contacted?
- Peer review. Did other authorities review the publication for quality?
- Updated Web pages. How old is the information?
- Citations. Where did the information come from?
- Tone of the report. Are claims exaggerated, unsubstantiated, or one-sided?

That being said, remain skeptical.

STEP TWO: NARROW THE CHOICE OF PROBLEMS

After you identify an important general problem (e.g., pressure ulcers among patients with spinal cord injuries) and conduct a literative search, gradually narrow the problem to one specific question that can be answered in one study. The reason is simple. A general problem is too broad and requires too many studies to solve in one instance. A good (specific) question can be answered in one study.

Imagine a general problem (such as pressure ulcers among patients with spinal cord injuries) at the beginning of a funnel along with all possible factors (variables) that can contribute to the development of pressure ulcers. These contributing factors may include diagnosis, activity level, sensation, humidity, shear forces, seating surface, body weight, nutrition, temperature, and age. It is not possible to study all of these factors in one study, but it may be possible to narrow the problem to a few of these factors. In this example, you may limit your choice to only one problem (pressure ulcers) among a particular group (persons with spinal cord injuries) who use a particular treatment approach (water cushions).

STEP THREE: DEVELOP A SPECIFIC QUESTION

WHAT IS A SPECIFIC QUESTION?

Toddlers often ask nonspecific, puzzling, one-word questions. Imagine a toddler walking up to you and saying, "Bath?" What does that mean? Does it mean "Do we have a bath?" "Is someone in the bath?" or "May I take a bath?" Certainly this youngster will need to elaborate before we know what he or she wants to know. One word is not sufficient.

Now imagine you are in a lecture hall filled with 500 students and one professor. You raise your hand and ask, "Prematurity?" The professor understandably looks puzzled and asks you to elaborate. On your next attempt, you ask, "Early intervention, prematurity?" The question (regarding early intervention in the care of premature infants) is still vague and too general. Finally, you try to focus (perhaps going to that fraternity party last night was not such a good idea after all) and blurt out, "What is the effect of early intervention on the motor development of premature infants?" Aha! Now you are beginning to ask a specific question, but it took more than one word.

WHAT ARE THESE THINGS CALLED VARIABLES?

In research, we want to understand things (*constructs* and *concepts,* such as heat, traction, pain, intelligence, or coordination). Specifically, we want to describe things, relate things, or determine the impact of some things on other things. To do this, we must assign values to these things so they can be measured. Once we convert them into *variables* that have two or more values, these things can be measured and therefore studied. They are called *variables* because they are things that change and have different values in the group. Some people have more of the variable, others have less of it. The amount varies (how much cancer, pain, coordination, intelligence; how many falls or treatments). Variables are located within a question. There are two types of variables—independent and dependent.[12]

Independent Variables (Predictors)

Independent variables can be thought of as intervention or treatments that are varied in the sense that some subjects may receive the treatment and others may not (the treatment can be manipulated).[1] Subjects can even be given different values of the treatment in terms of varying dosages (type of treatment, frequency, duration, intensity). Independent variables are sometimes called *predictors.* In this book, the term *treatment* is used instead of *independent variable* for the sake of simplicity.

Example: Ultrasound Treatments

Some groups may receive a high dosage (3.0 W/cm^2), some groups may receive an average dosage (1.5 W/cm^2), and some groups may receive no ultrasound at all (0 W/cm^2). Each group receives a different level of the treatment. It varies.

Dependent Variables (Criteria Measures, Response Variables)

Dependent variables are responses, outcomes, performances, or behaviors that may vary and that the investigator wishes to study, such as the amount of pain, range of motion, or skill level).[1] In an effort to study relationships in science, we try to determine whether a response in the dependent variable *depends on* the independent variable.[13]

Example: Pain

Not everyone in the population has pain or for that matter experiences the same amount of pain as everyone else. Some have more, some have less, and some have no pain at all. It varies.

Continuous versus Discrete Variables

Variables are described as either *discrete* or *continuous*. Continuous variables can have any value, such as 1 W or 1.00985 W. Discrete variables, on the other hand, cannot have a value less than 1. In other words, one can have 1 child or 2 children but not 1.5 children. Another example is pregnancy. Either you are or you are not pregnant—you cannot be half pregnant. So why is it important to know this? It is easier to detect smaller changes in continuous variables, which vary along a continuum, than changes in discrete variables, which are limited in the values they can assume. It may be helpful to use a staircase and escalator as metaphors for discrete and continuous variables, respectively (Figure 4-1).

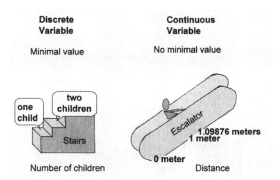

Figure 4-1. Think of discrete variables as values that can rest only on landings of a staircase and not between steps. Continuous variables, on the other hand, have no minimal value so they can stop at any point along an escalator.

ANATOMY OF THE QUESTION

Questions have a familiar format. Typically there are (1) a characteristic, relationship, or effect that the investigator wishes to study, (2) one or more variables, and (3) people who participate in the study. By reading across the following columns, and adding *to determine* or *what is (or are) the* to the beginning of the sentence, you have the basic format of a problem statement or research question.

Characteristic, Relationship, or Effect	Variable	Persons
The effect of	ultrasound on musculoskeletal pain	among dancers
The relationship between	age and falls	among elderly persons
The eating habits of	fatty foods	among cardiac patients
The frequency of	compression fractures	among patients with osteopenia
The incidence	of lung cancer	among female smokers

QUESTIONS EVOLVE AS THE KNOWLEDGE BASE GROWS

Our knowledge base helps determine the kind of question we pose. If we know little about a problem, then questions that *describe* the phenomenon may be warranted. After all, how can we study a group if we know nothing about them? Once we know more about a group, we need to ask questions to establish *associations*. Finally, if a large body of descriptive and associational knowledge already exists, it does not make sense to conduct yet another nonexperimental study in that area. Instead, an experiment, in which we seek to establish *causality* between some of the related variables, may be warranted.

DIFFERENT WAYS TO WRITE A QUESTION

Questions can be formulated into either a problem statement or a research question.

Problem Statements

Problem statements are questions posed during the study but are written in the form of a statement because the investigator has an expectation based on theory regarding the outcome of the study.[1,14] If the question is phrased in terms of a problem statement, the investigators usually tell readers about the expected outcome (research hypothesis). Frequently, the problem statement begins with words such as "To determine . . . "

Research Questions

Research questions are questions posed when the investigator does not have an expectation based on theory regarding the outcome of the study.[12,14] Hence the investigator does not offer a research hypotheses (or prediction). In reports of this type of research, the question frequently begins with words such as "What is the . . . ?"

MARRYING AND DIVORCING QUESTIONS

Finding a good question can be extremely difficult. For some graduate students, it is somewhat analogous to finding a soul mate, or at least a good marriage. Investigators may painfully go through several potential questions before the right one is identified. Like a bad but long-sustained marriage, it is not always easy to separate from a question in which one has invested a great deal of time. If the investigator becomes attached to a question that has no prospects of being answered, the question is best abandoned (divorced) and replaced with a question with better prospects. Finding that special question must meet certain requirements.

Finding Mr. or Ms. Right: The Requirements

The right research question must meet three "marital" requirements[1]—feasibility, importance, and answerability.

Feasibility. The solution to the question must be feasible. The investigator must have skill, laboratory space, support, equipment, accessibility to subjects, and money to answer the question successfully. If you need a federal budget and NASA technical support to complete a study, move onto the next question.

Importance. The question must be important enough to justify the expenditure of time and resources. If your question seems to put committee members to sleep, if the problem really is not very important, or if the problem already has been addressed, consider moving onto the next question.

Answerability

As discussed in Chapter 2, philosophical questions such as the meaning of life cannot be answered through the scientific method. If the phenomenon of interest cannot be measured, move onto the next question.[1]

COMMON MISTAKES WITH QUESTIONS

The "So What" Question

Perhaps the most devastating thing a person can say about your proposed research is, *"So what? Why is it important?"*[1] You should not take it personally. What they are really saying is that your question may not be clinically or theoretically important. For example, you may find sideways head movements performed by Middle Eastern

dancers fascinating and want to devote the rest of your life to its study. Although the question is interesting, it may not serve to solve a clinical problem or resolve a theoretical controversy. You cannot justify a study simply because it has never been done before or it has never been measured with your instrument. Always try to identify a clinical and theoretical need for your proposed study because you never know when someone will ask the "so what" question.

The Cart before the Horse Syndrome

Students often try to ask a question that can be answered with a measuring instrument to which they have convenient access. Students with this problem have a method in search of a question. In a sense, they are placing the cart before the horse (Figure 4-2). In life, a problem should stimulate formulation of a question. Finding a method (instrument and analysis) is a concern only after you have identified an important, feasible, and answerable question. Doing it the other way around often frustrates and prolongs graduate education because the student lacks a good question to drive a study.

The Shotgun Approach

Another common mistake in research is trying to measure every possible characteristic. This can be called the *shotgun approach* because you are trying to hit (study) everything in sight. For example, the student may wish to measure all aspects of gait for every joint in the body: velocity, step length, stride length, step time, cycle time, stance time, double support time, angular displacement, angular velocity, and angular acceleration. Most students cannot offer a rationale for measuring all those variables. Unacceptable excuses include (1) "The instrument provides those data" and (2) "I don't want to miss anything." Unless you are conducting an *exploratory study*,[15] in which the goal is to generate rather than test hypotheses, you need to have a reason for measuring things. The best reason for measuring something is always the same—to answer your question.

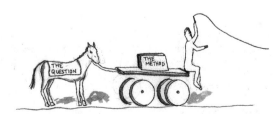

Figure 4-2. Student frequently suffers from cart before the horse syndrome and can spend months or years with a method in search of a question.

THINGS TO DO

1. Identify a potential question generated from the discussion or conclusion section of a research report. Authors frequently include recommendations for future studies.
2. Conduct a literature search of a topic of your choice using the following sources: (a) biomedical index (chose two), (b) government document index, (c) dissertation index, (d) statistical index, (e) press release, (f) current news story, and (g) textbook source.
3. Conduct a literature search using two different databases (use the same key words) to determine whether your results yield identical or different citations.
4. Examine a Web site during a literature search and evaluate the quality of the site on the basis of (a) source, (b) contact information, (c) peer review, (d) updated Web pages, (e) citations, and (f) tone of the report.
5. Identify a question from a report and determine whether it meets the requirements of a good question. Is it (a) important, (b) feasible, and (c) answerable? Pose your own question and determine whether it meets these requirements.
6. Identify two types of questions in a research report: (a) a research question (author does not have a hypothesis) and (b) a problem statement (author does have a hypothesis).
7. Identify a question in a research report and identify the (a) variables, (b) type of people studied (population), and (c) what is being studied (characteristic, relationship, or treatment effect).

REFERENCES

1. Portney LG, Watkins MP. *Foundations of Clinical Research: Applications to Practice.* Upper Saddle River, N.J.: Prentice Hall; 2000.
2. Nachmias CF, Nachmias D. *Research Methods in the Social Sciences.* 5th ed. New York: St. Martin's Press, 1996.
3. Degroot LJ, Siegler M. The morning-report syndrome and medical search. *N Engl J Med.* 1979;301: 1285–1287.
4. Kahn CR. Picking a research problem: the critical decision. *N Engl J Med.* 1994;330:1530–1533.
5. Schlein AM. *Find It Online: The Complete Guide to Online Research.* Tempe, Ariz: Facts on Demand Press; 1999.
6. Kimmel S. WWW tools in reference services. In: Diaz KR, ed. *Reference Sources on the Internet: Off the Shelf and onto the Web.* New York: Haworth Press; 1997:5–20.
7. Roper FW, Boorkman JA. *Introduction to Reference Sources in the Health Sciences.* 3rd ed. Metuchen, NJ: Medical Library Association; 1994:53–112.
8. Notess GR. *Government Information on the Internet.* 2nd ed. Lanham, Md: Bernan Press; 1998.
9. Dickersin K, Scherer R, Lefebvre C. Identifying relevant studies for systematic review. *BMJ.* 1994; 309:1286–1291.
10. Berinstein P. *Finding Statistics Online: How to Locate the Elusive Numbers You Need.* Medford, NJ: Information Today; 1998.
11. Maxwell B. *How to Find Health Information on the Internet.* Washington, DC: Congressional Quarterly; 1998.
12. Light RJ, Singer JD, Willett JB. *By Design: Planning Research on Higher Education.* Cambridge, Mass: Harvard University Press; 1990.
13. Schroeder LD, Sjoquist DL, Stephan PE. *Understanding Regression Analysis: An Introductory Guide.* Newbury Park, Calif: Sage Publications; 1986.
14. Roscoe JT. *Fundamental Research Statistics for the Behavioral Sciences.* New York: Holt, Rinehart & Winston; 1969.
15. Cohen J. Things I have learned (so far). *Am Psychol.* 1990;45:1304–1312.

5

Hypotheses

Once you have a question, you can make a claim (hypothesis) about the answer to the question.

WHAT ARE HYPOTHESES?

Hypotheses are claims, tentative answers, or predictions that reveal the investigator's expectation of the outcome of the study.[1]

TWO TYPES OF HYPOTHESES

There are two types of hypothesis—null and research.[2] Null hypotheses (statistical hypotheses) always are claims that no differences exist. A null hypothesis is required when claims are to be statistically tested. A research hypothesis (alternative hypothesis) tells readers what investigators think they will find. In research, if the null hypothesis (no difference is found) is rejected, the alternative, research hypothesis (the expected difference is found) is accepted.

The Null Hypothesis: There Is No Difference

The null hypothesis is a claim that no statistically significant differences or relationships exist between variables and that any differences are simply due to chance. Regardless of what the investigator believes, the null hypothesis is always the same. It is the claim that any outcome probably is due to chance and that therefore no real differences between groups or treatments can be expected at the end of the study.

Although it may seem a bit schizophrenic to ask a question and follow the question immediately with a tentative answer that no statistically significant results will be found, questions must be converted into null hypotheses to be tested statistically. In a sense, the null hypothesis is like our judicial system in that everyone is first assumed to be the innocent (no different from anyone else) unless they are proved guilty (different) with evidence.[3]

A hypothesis cannot be *proved* in one study because mistakes can always find their way into a study.[4,5] The study has to be replicated. Regard with caution claims that an author has proved something.

The Research (Alternative) Hypothesis: What I Think Will Happen

Research hypotheses tell readers what the investigator expects to find and commits the investigator to that expectation. Investigators cannot change their hypotheses after a study begins. The situation is like betting on a horse race. You cannot place your bet after the race starts. And you cannot collect your winnings unless you place a bet (commit to a particular outcome) *before* the race begins. The rationale for a research hypothesis usually is based on a theory. Christopher Columbus's research hypothesis was that by sailing west, he could reach the East. His hypothesis was based on the notion that the world was round.[6]

Although research hypotheses are more common in research reports than are null hypotheses, a null hypothesis is necessary to conduct a statistical test of significance.[4]

WHAT DO HYPOTHESES LOOK LIKE?

A hypothesis can be identified as a conditional prediction in the "if, then" portion of a sentence.[7] If treatment A is introduced, then reaction B will occur. A hypothesis also can be more formally stated as a proclamation: "There will or will not be a relationship." Regardless of the form of a hypothesis, the expected relationship among variables must be revealed. Examples are as follows.

When No Relationship Is Expected (Null Hypothesis)

There is no relationship between intelligence and shoe size among clinicians.

There is no significant difference in the success rate of patients treated by male clinicians and female clinicians.

When a Relationship Is Expected (Nondirectional Hypothesis)[2]

There is a relationship between sleep deprivation and examination grades in first-year medical students.

There is a significant difference in test scores between students who study all semester and students who cram the night before an examination.

When a Specific Relationship Is Expected (Directional Hypothesis)

There is an inverse relationship between sleep deprivation and examination grades in first-year medical students.

Students who study all semester score significantly *higher* on examinations than do students who cram the night before the examination.

The Research Question: I Have No Clue

If an investigator has a question but does not have any expectation of an outcome based on theory, you probably will not find a hypothesis stated in the study.[8] The area of research may be new, untapped, or require further exploration. Instead the investigator simply poses a research question.

What is the effect of sleep deprivation on examination performance among graduate students?

How Many Hypotheses Do You Need?

You need a sufficient number of hypotheses to answer your question. If for example, you want to determine the effect of a treatment on motor control among young and older persons, you may need three hypotheses to answer all questions. (1) The first hypothesis examines the effect of treatment on the motor control of the young group. (2) The second hypothesis examines the effect of treatment on the motor control of the older group. (3) The third hypothesis examines any differences in motor control between the young and the older group during the treatment. In other words, if you have two treatments (variables), you usually need three hypotheses: one hypothesis for each treatment and a third for the interaction.[2]

Readdressing the Hypotheses

Once you state a hypothesis, collect data, and test the hypothesis, you report whether the hypothesis was supported or not supported in the results section of a report. That is, you state whether your prediction regarding the outcome of the study was correct or incorrect. An author typically states that the particular null hypothesis is rejected or not rejected depending on the outcome.

COMMON MISTAKES WITH HYPOTHESES

Failing to State the Hypothesis before Data Collection

You must state your hypothesis *before* the experiment. If formulation of the hypothesis is influenced by the data (peeking at the data), the probability rules of statistical tests may no longer hold true.[9] Using the horse race metaphor, you would be hard-pressed to collect your winnings at the track if you placed your bet after the horse came in.

Failing to State a Directional Hypothesis When Theory Supports a Direction

It puzzles me that students spend a great deal of time predicting the outcome of the proposed study on the basis of a large body of theory and then state a null or nondirectional hypothesis. The research hypothesis is a statement of prediction guided by theory. If you have theory, use it!

Confusing Theory with Hypotheses

Theory and *hypotheses,* although often interchangeable in casual conversation, are distinct in meaning for researchers. A theory organizes information into a coherent, understandable whole and helps us predict future events. A hypothesis, on the other hand, is a tentative answer to questions we ask as we try to predict, on the basis of the investigator's theory, the outcome of a study.[10]

Confusing Knowledge with Hypotheses

Knowledge is derived from hypotheses (claims or predictions) that have been repeatedly tested and accepted (or not rejected) after well-controlled research. Many therapeutic interventions unfortunately are based on untested hypotheses that have not been confirmed (the clinician's practice is based on belief in what will happen) rather than established knowledge.[11] In other words, the clinician may simply state, "I predict it will work *in theory.*"

THINGS TO DO

1. Identify hypotheses in five research reports: (a) Are variables included and clearly related in the hypotheses? (b) Are null or research hypotheses stated? (c) How many hypotheses are stated? (d) Are there enough hypotheses to answer the question? (e) Are the hypotheses addressed later in the report, in the results section?

REFERENCES

1. Nachmias CF, Nachmias D. *Research Methods in the Social Sciences.* 5th ed. New York: St. Martin's Press; 1996.

2. Portney LG, Watkins MP. *Foundations of Clinical Research: Applications to Practice.* Upper Saddle River, N.J.: Prentice Hall; 2000.

3. Gehlbach SH. *Interpreting the Medical Literature.* 3rd ed. New York: McGraw-Hill; 1993.

4. Munro BH, Page EB. *Statistical Methods for Health Care Research.* 2nd ed. Philadelphia: JB Lippincott; 1993.

5. Angell M, Kassirer JP. Clinical research: what should the public believe? [Editorial.] *N Engl J Med.* 1994;331:189–190.

6. Beveridge WIB. *The Art of Scientific Investigation.* 3rd ed. New York: Vintage Books; 1957.

7. Hempel CG. *Philosophy of Natural Science.* Englewood Cliffs, N.J.: Prentice-Hall; 1966.

8. Light RJ, Singer JD, Willett JB. *By Design: Planning Research on Higher Education.* Cambridge, Mass: Harvard University Press; 1990.

9. Bailar JC III. Science, statistics, and deception. *Ann Intern Med.* 1986;104:259–260.

10. Rensberger B. *How the World Works: A Guide to Science's Greatest Discoveries.* New York: Quill William Morrow; 1986.

11. Dykes MHM. Uncritical thinking in medicine: the confusion between hypothesis and knowledge. *JAMA.* 1974;227:1275–1277.

6
Theory

Once you state your hypothesis (claim), you should tell the reader why you expect the findings to turn out as specified. In other words, state the theory that explains and predicts the anticipated outcome of the study.

WHAT IS THEORY?

Theory helps us make sense out of your research outcome and provides a richer understanding of the problem.[1]

THE LITERAL MEANING OF THEORY

The Greek root of *theory* is *thea,* which means "viewing."[2] It is also the root of *theater.* Hence, it may be easiest to think of theory in terms of its word origins. That is, imagine yourself at the theater, observing a play or concert and contemplating your experience of it (Figure 6-1). The visual and auditory inputs are data (information) that bombard your senses and makes an impression on you. Theory in research is like that. You look at your data after conducting a study and develop an impression of what they mean.

As human beings, we seem to have an innate need to make sense of things and to know when they are going to happen again.[3] Theory is useful in health professions because if we understand how a treatment works, we may be able to predict when or with what patients it will work in the future.[4] Equally important is that theory enables us to piece together seemingly unrelated observations into a meaningful whole that makes the world a more understandable place.

WHAT'S THE BIG DEAL ABOUT THEORY?

Theories are developed to help interpret the results of a study. You are presented with a puzzling observation and are trying to understand and explain it. That is a big

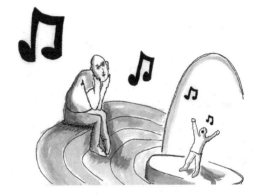

Figure 6-1. *Theory* and *theater* have the same root. You reflect on your data (the music) and develop an impression of its meaning.

deal. Instead of just knowing whether your treatment works, you want to know *how* it works. It works because . . . .

Example: Gravity

Observation: An Apple Drops from a Tree and Falls to the Ground.
Theory: An apple falls to the ground because of (or is explained by) some attractive force acting between the mass of the apple and the earth (i.e., law of gravity).
Hypothesis: If an apple should fall in the future, we predict it will accelerate at 9.8 m/s^2 toward the earth according to this law.

Example: Thunder

Observation: Thunder
Theory: Thunder occurs because lightning heats up the air, causing a quick expansion and contraction of air molecules, thus making sound waves.[5]
Hypothesis: If lightning should occur in the future, we should expect thunder.

THE CONFUSION ABOUT THEORY: THE JARGON

There is no one way to describe how the term *theory* is used in the literature. This ambiguity often leaves students perplexed and insecure at the mere mention of this six-letter word.[6] Scientists from different fields (e.g., biologists, social scientists, educators, and medical researchers) frequently use a wide array of terms when discussing theory. These terms include *classification, conceptual framework, theoretical framework, theoretical rationale, model, frame of reference,* or simply *framework.*

THEORY DEVELOPMENT

HOW ARE THEORIES CREATED?

Theories are created when ideas (concepts and constructs) are linked together to form principles that demonstrate the relationship between these ideas.[7] You can use the example of bones to gain a visual understanding of theory.

Example: Bones

Imagine that during a hike, you find seven bones. The bones look like cervical vertebrae (concept) and you try to determine whether they belong to the same animal. As you arrange the bones in size from large to small, you find that the bones (data) fit together perfectly (a postulate or principle demonstrating that the bones are related). The relationship of seven bones suggests they came from the same animal and that the animal most likely is a mammal because mammals with few exceptions have only seven cervical vertebrae.[8]

Now imagine that you find an eighth cervical bone that fits perfectly behind the seventh. You now have to *revise* your theory about the type of animal because mammals typically have only seven cervical vertebrae. Because your original theory no longer explains the new datum (the eighth vertebrae), you conclude the bones probably belong to a different kind of animal, which has additional neck bones.

TWO STRATEGIES FOR CREATING THEORIES

Theories are created by means of either (1) noticing an important pattern in a set of *observations* or (2) having an imaginative *insight* into how the world probably works.[2] Darwin's theory of evolution was the result of his noticing patterns in the collected evidence of bird anatomy (beak size and shape) and island diet.[6] On the other hand, Einstein's theory of relativity was based more on imaginative insight into how the universe works. Einstein is said to have been riding a streetcar in Bern when he realized that stationary and moving clocks may not run at the same rate.[3] Who said commuting is a waste of time?

WHO CREATES THEORY?

Anyone can create or espouse a theory—you, I, or a person on the street. You don't need a doctorate, a license, or permission from the government. What's important is that the theory be useful in explaining reality.

HOW WELL CAN A THEORY EXPLAIN REALITY?

Theories vary in their ability to explain things. Theories may explain a great deal, little, or nothing at all. Theories also may be well developed, sometimes incorporating other earlier theories to explain almost everything about a subject, or be poorly developed and explain very little.

Theories do not necessarily have to be correct at all to qualify as a theory. In other words, theories may be bizarre and baseless (invalid) or may be supported by scientific studies (valid) and well accepted by the scientific community.

Good theories offer the most comprehensible explanation of existing observations and facts. For example, Newton incorporated Kepler's theory of planetary motion and Galileo's theory of falling bodies into his theory of gravity. In other words, Newton's theory of gravity explains both Kepler's observations in astronomy and Galileo's observations in physics, placing both of them under one roof[3] (Figure 6-2).

HOW WELL DEVELOPED IS THE THEORY?

The following terms relate to how well developed a theory is in explaining something. The meanings may be used somewhat differently in different disciplines.[4]

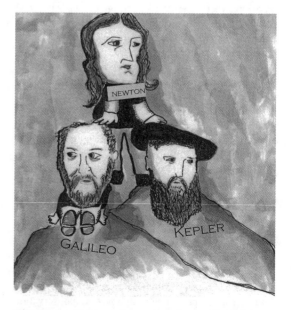

Figure 6-2.   Newton, who stood on the shoulders of giants (Galileo and Kepler), built upon their knowledge base.

Taxonomy

Taxonomy is an early development of a theory whereby ideas are organized and categorized. The periodic table is a classic example of taxonomy. In my opinion however, the periodic table is much more than a system of classification, because it not only organizes information (the table) but historically predicted the characteristics of elements not yet discovered.

The Periodic Law.   Mendeleyev, who discovered the periodic law while preparing a textbook for his chemistry course, organized the known elements in life according to atomic weight. In doing so, he noticed that elements had a repeating (periodic) pattern of properties as atomic weight increased. When he organized the elements into families with similar properties, he noticed gaps in the table. Because he knew where the gaps were, he could accurately predict that undiscovered elements with associated properties would fill the gaps.

Mendeleyev stated ". . . we must expect the discovery of many elements that are still unknown to us, such as elements similar to Al and Si, which would occupy the space between atomic weights 65 to 75."[9(p36)] Fourteen years later, germanium (atomic weight 72.6) was discovered and closely matched the predicted properties of the missing element. In summary, the story of the periodic table is a good example of how theory can both organize and predict phenomena.[9]

Frameworks

Frameworks are structures or schemes.[10] Conceptual frameworks begin to provide a structure for organizing and relating ideas (concepts).[4,11]

Theory

Theory is considered a more highly developed framework of related ideas to provide more explanation and to allow predictions based on the organization of ideas (concepts) in the framework (related terms include *theoretical rationale* and *theoretical framework*).[4]

Models.   Models are a way to simplify and more easily understand a theory by drawing a picture of it. Someone may say, "What's your model?" If you are explaining a theory you may verbalize it and then point to a model and say, "It looks like this."[6] A model makes a theory more concrete and understandable, often with visual aids. For example, the relationship between planetary orbits often is demonstrated in the classroom with a model in which Ping-Pong balls, the planets, are located at specified distances from a larger ball that represents the sun. In an attempt to teach the difficult notion of the stretch reflex in a therapeutic exercise course, I constructed a model of a stretch reflex with wood, springs, light-emitting diodes, and buzzers.[12]

Laws

Laws are highly developed theories that can accurately predict outcomes, often under various situations.

THEORIES ARE TEMPORARY EXPLANATIONS

Theories are developed to provide the best *current* explanation of reality on the basis of existing information. When new information becomes available, new theories have to be proposed or existing theories have to be modified (changed) to accommodate and explain this growing knowledge base.[1,2,7,13] Thus theories are only temporary explanations of reality.

IS YOUR THEORY USEFUL?

Once you have developed a theory, you need to know whether it is useful. Although many theories have been espoused to explain some aspect of reality, not all theories are useful. It may not be possible to verify the theory through testing (hypothesis testing). A useful theory can be verified through experimentation. In a sense, the theory of creation—that the world was created in 7 days—is not useful because it is impossible for scientists to verify it through experimentation: we can't interview the creator.

THEORY TESTING (TESTING THE HYPOTHESIS)

To test a theory, make a prediction (hypothesis) based on your theory, and test the prediction through experimentation to determine whether what you predicted does occur. Technically, you are testing the hypothesis to determine the validity of the theory. You want to determine whether there is a match (or fit) between your prediction (the hypothesis) and reality (the data from your study). It has been said that much of what scientists do all their lives is hypothesis testing. So that you are not accused of perverting the language of science, make sure you say "hypothesis testing" rather than "theory testing" when conversing with "men and women of science."

HYPOTHESIS TESTING AND THE CLINICIAN

The notion of hypothesis testing should not be new to clinicians because they engage in it every time they reevaluated a patient after treatment. Does the outcome match the expectation of how the patient should have responded to the treatment on the basis of an understanding of what the treatment is supposed to do?[1] If the treatment was pool therapy, you would expect a weak, obese patient to walk with less effort in the pool than out of the pool because theory (Archimedes' principle) tells you as much. The message to clinicians is that you are testing hypotheses with your patients in the clinic every day. You probably were just calling it something else.

Example: Moon Made of Cheese

Your Prediction of Reality.   You want a more accurate description of the composition of the moon. Is it made of cheese? You claim or predict that the moon is made of cheese (your hypothesis).

Your Reason for the Prediction.   On what did you base your prediction? What is your theory? Why cheese and not plain rock? Perhaps you have documentation that a Swiss cheese company made a secret mission to the moon thousands of years ago and you believe the presence of the Swiss on the moon has somehow altered its surface composition, which now resembles holes characteristic of Swiss cheese. Granted, your theory is bizarre but it's your theory, and it led you to develop your prediction.

Test Your Prediction.   Now it's time to test your prediction. That is, run a study and collect evidence (data) to see whether your prediction is correct or incorrect. In this example, your study involves going to the moon (a very expensive study) and collecting material on the surface to see if it is made of cheese (the evidence).

Does Your Prediction of Reality Match the True Reality?   The investigator needs to determine whether his or her claims of reality (hypotheses) match the reality provided by evidence.[6] Imagine the researcher's hypothesis (imagined reality) and reality (data from the study) as shapes. By conducting a study, you determine whether these two realties are congruent, that is, whether they fit or match each other (Figure 6-3).

If Your Prediction Is Correct.   If your hypothesis of a cheesy moon is supported by the evidence, your prediction or expectation is correct. Your hypothesis is supported by evidence, and your theory is supported. Technically, your theory is not disconfirmed. In other words, your theory continues to be a possible explanation for reality because the evidence matches the expectation based on your theory.

If Your Prediction Is Incorrect.   If your hypothesis of a cheesy moon is not supported by the evidence, your prediction is incorrect, and your theory is disconfirmed. That is, your theory does not appear to be a possible explanation of reality because the evidence (cheeseless rock) does not match the expectation based on your theory. In other words, the theory is not a valid explanation of reality and should be discarded or modified. Perhaps the Swiss cheese company never visited the moon, or if they did visit, they apparently did not alter the surface.

Disconfirming Theories: The Shooting Gallery

Strangely, in the language of science, experiments try to disconfirm rather than confirm theories. We would have to test a theory under many conditions to confirm that a particular theory is the correct one. Instead, we typically can only determine whether the theory being tested does

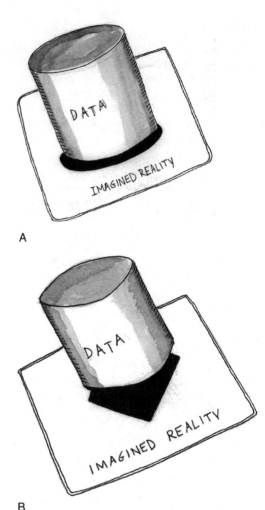

A

B

Figure 6-3.   (A) Theory is not disconfirmed when data continue to fit the imagined reality. (B) Theory is disconfirmed when data fail to fit the imagined reality.

not hold up under a particular condition, thus disconfirming it.[1,14]

What we are actually doing during an experiment is "shooting down" theories that do not agree with the data. These theories are dismissed from further consideration. You can imagine shooting down targets at a shooting gallery where each target represents a theory (Figure 6-4). Theories that continue to be supported by experimental data and remain standing, continue to be possible explanations for reality (valid theories) until research disconfirms them.

THEORY: HISTORICAL EXAMPLES

It may be useful to consolidate your understanding of theory with some classic examples from history.

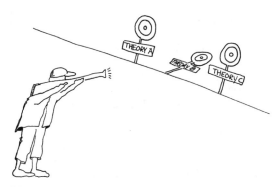

Figure 6-4. Disconfirming a theory—targets in a shooting gallery—can be likened to shooting down theories that are not supported by the data.

THE CIRCULATION OF BLOOD

Blood originally was believed to ebb and flow to and from the heart rather than circulate in one direction and return to the heart. William Harvey reasoned that too much blood was being pumped through the heart every hour for it not to be circulating. He found evidence of one-way valves in veins to suggest a unidirectionality of blood and inferred that a network not visible to the naked eye must connect arteries to veins to close the loop and recirculate the blood.[15] Malpighi, using a microscope, later demonstrated the capillary system that Harvey predicted.[15–17]

MALARIA (BAD AIR)

Two theories were developed to explain the sickness among those who worked on the Panama Canal. The first theory, advanced by the contagions, was that the sickness was caused by contact. A second theory, advanced by the anticontagions, was that sickness was caused by bad air. Interestingly, neither theory was correct in predicting malaria. The disease was caused by parasites carried in the blood of mosquitoes (the worker would become sick once bitten by the insect). Ross Ronald found evidence of the parasite that caused malaria in the internal organs of mosquitoes. Hence, a "blood-transmitted" theory correctly predicted the sickness.[17]

HEADLESS WALKING CHICKENS

Beheaded chickens may continue to walk for a brief period before they die. This observation suggests that the brain is not critical for expressing the basic pattern of walking because once the head and brain are removed, walking continues. The theory called the *central pattern generator theory*, suggests that the mechanism responsible for the pattern of walking resides within the spinal cord.[18] Evidence of this theory can be found among both animals and humans with spinal cord lesions who can still demonstrate

a walking pattern on a moving treadmill if supported by a harness. In other words, the walking pattern is expressed despite a lack of descending supraspinal output.

EVOLUTION

Darwin asked why diversity existed in life. He observed a variety of adaptive features among birds (different sizes and shapes of beaks) and in different bird diets. He noticed that birds' beaks were curiously adapted to the birds' available food, suggesting that adaptations may favor survival of a species.[6]

ADAM'S TWELFTH RIB

Galen, a physician and authority on medicine in ancient Rome, stated that men had one fewer rib than women. This notion probably had biblical origins. Andreas Vesalius, one of the first to dissect human cadavers, disconfirmed this notion when he dissected and found all 12 ribs in men.[17]

COLUMBUS AND THE WEST

Columbus believed that by sailing west one would reach the Orient.[16] He based this hypothesis on the theory that the world was round (continuous) and not flat. Interestingly, Columbus incorrectly maintained that his hypothesis was correct on the basis of misinterpretation of his data. He did not actually reach the East as believed but instead found the New World in the West.

COMMON MISTAKES IN THINKING ABOUT RESEARCH

BIG AND SMALL PICTURES

Students frequently see the small picture in research (Does my treatment work?), but miss the big picture concerning *how* the treatment works so one can predict when these effects will occur again (explain the mechanism or theory behind the treatment).

THINGS TO DO

1. Identify a theory in your field and state how it was developed. What data (studies), clinical observations, or insights lead to the creation and development of the theory?
2. Identify a theory in your field and state whether it has been tested. In other words, what research has been conducted to determine whether the theory is valid?

REFERENCES

1. Portney LG, Watkins MP. *Foundations of Clinical Research: Applications to Practice.* Upper Saddle River, N.J.: Prentice Hall; 2000.
2. Tammivaara J, Shepard KF. Theory: the guide to clinical practice and research. *Phys Ther.* 1990;70:578–582.
3. Hazen RM, Trefil J. *Science Matters: Achieving Scientific Literacy.* New York: Doubleday; 1991.
4. Nachmias CF, Nachmias D. *Research Methods in the Social Sciences.* 5th ed. New York: St. Martin's Press; 1996.
5. Williams J. *USA Today: The Weather Book—An Easy to Understand Guide to the USA's Weather.* New York: Vintage Books; 1992.
6. Giere RN. *Understanding Scientific Reasoning.* 4th ed. Fort Worth, Tex: Harcourt Brace College; 1997.
7. Payton OD. *Research: The Validation of Clinical Practice.* Philadelphia: FA Davis; 1979.
8. Webster D, Webster M. *Comparative Vertebrate Morphology.* New York: Academic Press; 1974.
9. Kelman P, Stone AH. *Mendeleyev: Prophet of Chemical Elements.* Englewood, N.J.: Prentice Hall; 1970.
10. *Webster's New International Dictionary.* 3rd ed., s.v. "framework."
11. Mosey AC. *Applied Scientific Inquiry in the Health Professions: An Epistemological Orientation.* 2nd ed. Bethesda, Md: American Occupational Therapy Association; 1996.
12. Batavia M, McDonough AL. Demonstrating the stretch reflex: a mechanical model. *Am Biol Teacher.* 2000;62(7).
13. Etzioal A. Understanding of science. *Science.* 1972;177:391.
14. Campbell DT, Stanley JC. *Experimental and Quasi-experimental Designs for Research.* Boston: Houghton Mifflin; 1963.
15. Hart MH. *The 100: A Ranking of the Most Influential Persons in History.* Secaucus, NJ: Citadel Press; 1987.
16. Beveridge WIB. *The Art of Scientific Investigation.* 3rd ed. New York: Vintage Books; 1957.
17. *Random House Webster's Dictionary of Scientists.* New York: Random House; 1997.
18. Peterson I. *The Jungle of Randomness: A Mathematical Safari.* New York: John Wiley & Sons; 1998.

7

Designs

Once you identify a question, provide a tentative prediction (hypothesis) about the outcome, and justify the prediction with theory, you need to plan or design the study.

WHAT ARE DESIGNS?

The design is a plan for a study that will enable you to test your hypothesis. It is the blueprint[1] that will guide you through your problem to the answer to your question. In a team-sports metaphor, the design helps answer the following questions: How many teams or individuals are playing? How are they selected? How long does the game last? How often is the score kept (i.e., How often are measurements taken?).

GOOD DESIGNS STRENGTHEN A STUDY

The ultimate purpose of any research endeavor that involves a question is to answer the question in a believable way. By choosing the correct design, you are protecting or vaccinating your study against mistakes that could otherwise undermine the study and make it less believable to the scientific community.

DESIGNS IN EVERYDAY LIFE

There are many types of research design, each of which serves a special purpose. It may be easiest to understand the concept of research design by first looking at more common, everyday examples of designs for shelters and vessels.

DESIGNS FOR SHELTERS

Each type of shelter is designed for a specific function and has its advantages and disadvantages. There is no perfect shelter to fill every purpose in life.

Small Tents

Small tents are designed to be lightweight for hiking, to protect campers from rain, and to sleep one or two people. They are not designed to protect against cold weather or to accommodate a large number of persons.

Circus Tents

Circus tents are huge tents designed to protect against rain, accommodate large crowds of spectators and animals, and provide an arena for entertainment.

Skyscrapers

Skyscrapers are tall buildings designed to provide a maximal amount of office or living space on a small plot of land.

DESIGNS FOR VESSELS

Vessels also have varied functions and designs.

Canoes

Canoes are small, narrow boats powered by one or two persons using paddles. They are designed for negotiating small bodies of water such as streams, lakes, and ponds. Canoes are not designed for transatlantic voyages.

Rowboats

Rowboats are small boats powered by a person or persons using oars. Because two persons can sit side-by-side, this is a good boat design for lovers. Like canoes, rowboats are not designed for long-distance travel.

Ocean Liners

Ocean liners and cruise ships are huge, sleep hundreds of people, can withstand the transatlantic travel, and usually offer entertainment. They are too large for travel in narrow waterways and too expensive to sail with only a few guests aboard.

RESEARCH DESIGNS

Like shelter and water travel, research offers many designs, each serving a different purpose. If the correct research design is chosen, it can protect the study from flaws (mistakes), making the findings of the study more believable. If the wrong research design is chosen for a particular question, the study becomes more vulnerable to flaws, rendering findings less believable. Choosing an appropriate research design can help vaccinate your study from becoming sick. Choose wisely.

A HISTORICAL NOTE ON RESEARCH METHODS: QUALITATIVE VERSUS QUANTITATIVE

There are almost as many ways to describe research as there are ways to slice a pie. Historically, it may be useful to view medical research as either qualitative (describing) or quantitative (counting).[2] *Qualitative methods* came first and have origins in the case report. In ancient Greece, Hippocrates described the fits of a child that caused disability. During Victorian times, Gull described anorexia, Osler described a child with cerebral palsy, and Charcot wrote on the hemianopia of a draper who after "recovering" from hemiplegia, could not resume a game of billiards because his visual field was lost on the right side. Even medical training initially relied on qualitative information such as learning to differentiate a normal heart sound from a murmur. *Quantitative methods* began with measurement of body temperature and growth and later became popular with the advent of diagnostic and interventional studies.[2]

TYPES OF RESEARCH DESIGN

There a two basic categories of research design—nonexperimental (descriptive, correlational) and experimental (experimental, quasiexperimental). Nonexperimental designs are meant to answer questions that have to do with describing things (e.g., What are the characteristics of smokers?) or how characteristics are related (e.g., Is smoking related to lung cancer?). The key point is that the investigator is an observer (a bystander[3]) in the study and does not actively intervene.

Experimental designs are meant to answer questions about causality (e.g., Does smoking cause lung cancer?). The key point is that the investigator is more than simply an observer in the study and actively manipulates the variables (treatments) to establish causality.[3] Experimental designs offer the strongest protection against mistakes for demonstrating cause-and-effect relationships. Although there is an abundance of designs,[4] only the most practical and popular designs in medicine, rehabilitation, and education are reviewed herein (see Appendix A for in-depth resources on design).

WHICH DESIGN IS BEST?

The type of design you choose depends on your question. Each research design has its own strengths and weaknesses[5] just as different shelter designs have advantages and limitations. A nonexperimental descriptive design is fine to describe the characteristics of a group but would be inappropriate to demonstrate cause and effect. An experimental design, although appropriate for demonstrating efficacy of treatment (cause and effect), is overkill if you simply want to describe something. A nonexperimental, epidemiologic study may be most fitting to identify risk factors and rare side effects. A qualitative study may be most appropriate to document one patient's experiences. In short, *choose the design that can best answer your question.*[6] Figure 7-1 is an algorithm of some common designs in research.

NONEXPERIMENTAL DESIGNS

Descriptive Studies

Descriptive designs are used to describe. Describe what? Characteristics, behaviors, attitudes, aptitudes, even a movement pattern. They are called *nonexperimental* because you are observing, not manipulating, the environment. This type of research usually is conducted before an experiment is performed. In a sense, you are starting to acquire information about a population (Figure 7-2).

Example

You travel in a space ship to the planet Krypton and discover a whole community of supermen. As a first step in research, you may want to describe this group of people. You may find, for instance, that they all wear red capes, are faster than a speeding bullet, and are more powerful than a locomotive (we won't mention the tights). You use a nonexperimental design because you are describing this interesting group of people. You record your observations accurately.

How Much Control Is There? Descriptive designs offer the least control over variables in a study that may obscure the true nature of a phenomenon. In descriptive studies investigators nevertheless have to use good research practices to believably describe a group or issue. In other words, you need a carefully selected population, involve an unbiased investigator, and employ valid measurements.

When Are They Used? Descriptive designs are a good way to start if you don't know anything about a subject or problem. You can observe behaviors and characteristics and then explore and develop theories that may explain these observations.

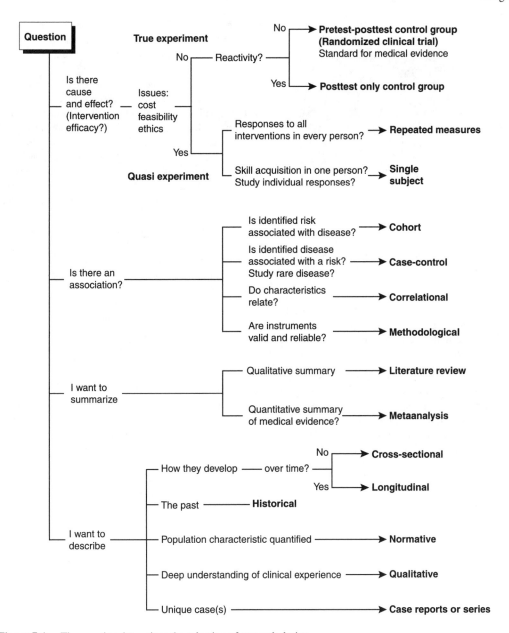

Figure 7-1. The question determines the selection of research design.

Types of Descriptive Studies

CASE REPORT OR CASE STUDY. A case report is a good means of bringing attention to an unusual case,[7–9] exploring possible mechanisms (theory) of a phenomenon,[10] and generating hypotheses.[11] In other words, vignettes[11] and anecdotes can alert the reader to an unsuspected association that can serve as the basis for future confirmatory designs. The case report is an appropriate choice whenever an investigator approaches a relatively unknown area in clinical care.[9]

Advantages of case reports include low cost, minimal ethical considerations (you are not withholding or manipulating treatment), and convenience (data usually have been collected during the course of treatment). The main disadvantage is that case reports have limited scientific merit (no ability to draw conclusions of causality).[11] In summary, case reports are exploratory rather than confirmatory and emphasize discovery over proof [9] (see Chapter 23).

Lashley provided a classic example of a case report in 1917 when he described a man who sustained a gunshot wound to the spinal cord and lost sensation to the leg although he was able to perform accurate leg movements. From this study, the notion of a *motor program* was born whereby the nervous system may not require sensory

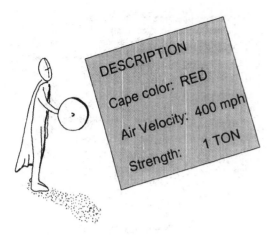

Figure 7-2. Descriptive designs provide information on the characteristics of a group, such as strength, height, and even cape size.

input for the control of movement.[10] The psychoanalytic theory of psychopathology, as developed by Freud, is another classic example in the use of case reports to generate theory.[9]

CASE SERIES.   A case series is used to describe the characteristics of several persons. Case series are a good way to bring attention to something unusual. The evidence is strengthened with several examples (cases) that support the observation. Cases can document exceptions to a rule, the usual course of a disease, or the feasibility of a therapy regardless of its true effectiveness.[3] The advantages and disadvantages of case series are similar to those of case reports.

In 1981, Hymes[8] provided a historic account of eight homosexual men who had a type of cancer usually found only among older persons. This case series became one of the first accounts of AIDS. In 1817, Parkinson provided a report of six persons with what he described as a "shaking palsy." Patients who fit this description later were referred to as having Parkinson's disease.[7]

DEVELOPMENTAL STUDIES
Cross-sectional Studies. Cross-sectional studies are indicated if you want to describe the typical developmental characteristics of different groups of individuals at various stages of life (e.g., describing the walking ability among groups of infants, young adults, and elderly adults).[12]

Longitudinal Studies. Longitudinal studies are indicated if you want to study a pattern of change over time (i.e., describe the development of a person or group's gait). Examples include Piaget's seminal observations of the cognitive development of children[13] and McGraw's classic observations of the motor development of twins.[14]

NORMATIVE RESEARCH.   Normative research is indicated if you want to describe quantitative characteristics of a particular population and how much these characteristics vary (e.g., record body weight and head circumference percentiles of infants from 0 to 8 years).[12,15]

QUALITATIVE RESEARCH.   The goal in qualitative studies is to achieve a deep understanding of a clinical matter. Qualitative research generally is aimed at understanding reality from the subject's point of view[12] and attempts to develop theory based on the data. One may describe the experiences of a person or group, such as a patient's perceptions during recovery from an illness or about a health care issue. The description by a Harvard-trained lawyer with quadriplegia of his frustration securing funds for a wheelchair under managed care provides a greater depth of insight into the issue than does quantitative analysis.[16] Despite its nonquantitative approach, qualitative research still has to be concerned with objective, unbiased, and believable methods of collecting data.[17]

Contrasting Qualitative with Quantitative Studies. Qualitative studies ask questions related to *what* rather than *how many.* Methods and analyses involve observation and interviews, usually with multiple methods and independent analysis by another researcher, to classify phenomena. In qualitative studies, the goal, which is inductive, is *to develop a theory* that is well-grounded in data.

Quantitative methods, in contrast, rely more on experimentation or correlational designs to count and statistically analyze phenomena. Quantitative goals are deductive and often involve *testing a theory* or, more correctly, testing a hypothesis that is based on theory.

Interestingly, qualitative studies are iterative and closed loop in that the method and hypothesis can change as data are collected and the study progresses to support an emerging theory. Quantitative approaches, on the other hand, are linear and open looped. The hypothesis and method are established before data collection and cannot be altered once the study begins.[18,19]

HISTORICAL RESEARCH.   Historical research is indicated if you want to describe something that happened in the past (e.g., describing the historical development of a health profession). Understanding what happened in the past may help clarify how conditions evolved to the present. Data are limited to surviving documents and interviews.[12] Future generations of researchers will no doubt examine the development of the clinical doctorate in physical therapy (DPT) that is currently underway.

SECONDARY ANALYSIS.   Secondary analysis involves reexamining existing data and perhaps testing new hypotheses with these data. The advantages are no data collection, minimal expense, and quick results concerning your question because the data are readily available. The disadvantage is that you do not know how credible the data are because you did not collect them.[12]

SUMMARIES. Literature reviews are useful to provide a qualitative, perhaps subjective, summary of a body of knowledge. Metaanalysis, on the other hand, offers a quantitative summary of medical evidence and can assist in establishing clinical guidelines. Decision analysis assesses the value of different management options in patient care. Economic analysis is used (i.e., cost to benefit ratio or cost-effectiveness analysis) to examine the financial issues related to a clinical problem.

Correlational Designs

In correlational designs, you are attempting to describe something, but you go one step farther to analyze whether a relationship or pattern exists among the things you are describing. Correlational designs offer greater controls over threats to internal validity than descriptive designs but less control than experimental designs. A relationship established with a correlational design can later be tested with an experimental design to determine causation.

Example

In the superman example, you may wonder whether there is a relationship between strength and kryptonite (a poison). You then use a correlational design to determine whether strength decreases as amount of exposure to kryptonite increases. You can measure amount of strength and kryptonite to confirm the existence of the pattern between the two that you predicted (Figure 7-3).

When Are They Used? Correlational designs are used when you want to determine the presence of an association between two variables. You cannot determine a cause-and-effect relationship with this design. For example, you can only determine whether persons who jog more frequently also have a higher prevalence of arthritis of the knee than do persons who do not. You cannot use this design to determine whether jogging causes arthritis.

How Much Control Is There? In addition to using good research practices in descriptive designs, the investigator also needs to choose an appropriate statistical

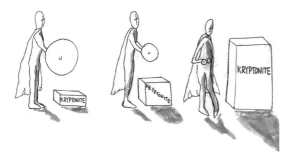

Figure 7-3. Correlational designs seek to establish associations such as the interdependence of strength and poison (kryptonite). The more poison there is, the less strength there is.

analysis to answer questions about associations in a believable manner.

Types of Correlational Studies

CROSS-SECTIONAL STUDIES. Cross-sectional studies are conducted to examine relationships at one point in time. For example, you want to examine the relationship between resting blood pressure and exercise habits. First you observe both resting blood pressure and exercise habits for a group of individuals. You then note any pattern or association between the two variables. You may notice that those who exercise more also have lower resting blood pressures. The two behaviors are related.

VALIDITY AND RELIABILITY STUDIES. The development and testing of a new measuring instrument is called *methodological research*[12] and frequently involves conducting validity and reliability studies to detemine whether new or untested instruments are accurate and reliable. You measure a range of values with an instrument (e.g., a bathroom scale) and determine whether you consistently obtain the same measurements with the same instrument (reliability study) or with a well-accepted, accurate instrument (validity study). For a clinical example, you may want to compare the accuracy of joint angles derived from goniometric measurements and from radiographs (a more accurate method) of the same joints (criterion validity study). These studies help establish confidence in your measuring instrument.

COHORT STUDIES. Cohort studies (longitudinal, follow-up studies)[11] are used to examine the association between a risk factor (now) and the development of a disease (later).[3] In these common epidemiologic studies, you may want to identify a risk factor now (smoking) and then determine whether smokers but not nonsmokers contract disease in the future. The advantage of this prospective study is that you observe people in their natural settings (they choose to smoke) because it is not ethical to make people smoke if you think it may harm them. Cohort studies, however, have a weaker degree of control over threats to internal validity than do experimental designs and therefore the results are not strong evidence of cause and effect. Longitudinal studies also can be expensive.[11]

CASE-CONTROL STUDIES. Case-control studies examine the association between a disease (now) and risk factors that can be uncovered from the past. *Case* refers to subjects who already have the disease[3] and *control* to those who do not. In these common epidemiologic studies, you may want to identify persons with and those without cancer to determine through records whether only those with the disease had been exposed to a risk factor such as smoking.

Case-control studies, which are retrospective, offer a weaker degree of control than do cohort studies, which are prospective. Case-control studies therefore are used to explore relationships until more rigorous designs can be implemented. A case-control study is considered convenient (patients already have the disease), efficient (data collection involves a review of records), and useful in the study of rare diseases.[3]

EXPERIMENTAL DESIGNS

In experimental and quasiexperimental designs, you are trying to determine the effect of one thing on something else, rather than describing or simply associating things. The key to these designs is that you are not only observing but also are actively intervening in the study by manipulating the independent variable. You may expose only one (experimental) group to the treatment and withhold it from the other (control) group to see whether the treatment (independent variable) has an effect on the outcome (dependent variable).

Example

In the superman example, you want to determine whether kryptonite, and only kryptonite reduces superpowers. To do this, you need to prevent the supermen from being exposed to other poisons, such as mercury, during the study. Experimental designs help you to determine the effect of one thing (kryptonite) on another (superpowers) while controlling for or preventing other possible causes (mercury) from having an effect during the study (Figure 7-4).

When Are They Used?

Experimental and quasiexperimental designs are used to establish causality.

How Much Control Is There?

Experimental and quasiexperimental designs offer strong protection (control) from threats to internal validity (i.e., extraneous, confounding variables) so you can confidently conclude that the treatment (independent variable) had an effect on the outcome (dependent variable). Exper-

imental designs offer even greater protection than quasi-experimental designs and are therefore the premier designs for determining cause-and-effect relationships. The randomized clinical trial (RTC) is an example of an experimental design that is the standard for testing the effectiveness of medical treatment.[11]

In addition to the same good research practices used in descriptive and correlational designs, experimental and quasiexperimental designs must include methods to avoid many potential mistakes (i.e., history, maturation, instrumentation, sampling error, regression to the mean, reactivity to instrumentation, and response sensitivity) to establish a cause-and-effect link in a credible manner. Potential mistakes are discussed in Part III.

Classification of Experimental Studies

Experimental and quasiexperimental designs can be described in two ways. The first classification is factorial design. The second classification is based on whether conditions are varied between subjects or within-subjects. Note that experimental and quasiexperimental designs are sometimes notated in the literature with Xs and Os. The X represents a group's exposure to an experimental treatment; the O represents a measurement, such as a pretest and posttest prior to and following an X (i.e., OXO).[4]

Factorial Design.   *Factorial design* refers to the number of treatments (factors, independent variables) included in a study. In a study with a one-way or single factor design, only one factor or treatment is examined. That factor can have more than one level (e.g., dosage) (Figure 7-5). For example, if the factor is a medication for Parkinson's disease, two levels can include no medication (0 mg) and medication (x mg). Three levels (dosages) may include no medication (0 mg), a low dose of medication (x mg), and a high dose of medication ($2x$ mg). A two-way factorial design can be used to examine two treatments and how they interact, such as medication and physical therapy (Figure 7-6). A three-way factorial design is used to examine three treatments, such as medication, physical therapy, and family support, and their interactions. For each factor (treatment), subjects may be exposed to various levels (dosages).

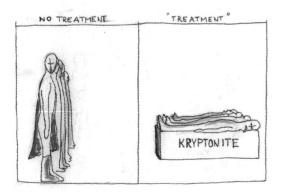

Figure 7-4.   Experimental designs seek to establish causality, such as the deleterious effects of poison (kryptonite) on superbeings.

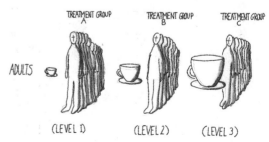

Figure 7-5.   Single factor designs are used to examine the effect of one treatment on an outcome. In this example, the treatment is coffee.

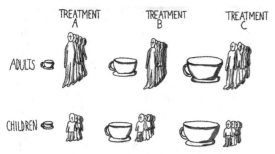

Figure 7-6. Factorial designs are used to examine the effect of more than one treatment or group membership on an outcome. In this example, two groups are examined: adults and children.

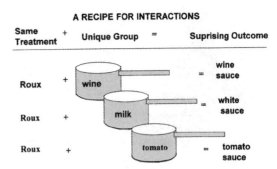

Figure 7-7. The cooking metaphor. Interactions between the identical "treatments" (roux) and different "patient populations" (wine, milk, and tomato) can have some unexpected outcomes.

INTERACTIONS: THE COMBINED EFFECT OF TWO TREATMENTS (INDEPENDENT VARIABLES). Examining the combined effect of more than one treatment on an outcome allows you to study interactions. Studying interactions makes sense because most events in life do not occur in isolation but occur in the presence of other events. Hence, multifactorial designs (designs with more than one independent variable) improve one's ability to generalize the findings to real life (external validity). When two events occur or treatments are administered together, the effect may be different from that of one or the other when observed for effectiveness alone.

Perhaps some of the most publicized interactions are those found on the back label of medications. Although sleeping pills can help you to sleep better and a little alcohol can make you feel better, the combination of alcohol and sleeping pills can kill you—a unique reaction what does not occur when either medication is taken alone in the proper dosage. It is important to examine the effects of interaction because not all patients respond to a treatment in the same manner. The treatment may work for some groups of patients but not for others.

Example: Cooking

Imagine studying three groups of people who are represented metaphorically as milk, tomato, and wine (Figure 7-7). Now you, the investigator would like to see the effect of a roux (treatment) (roux is a mixture of butter and flour) on the three groups. As you add the treatment (roux) to each group, you find that the three groups respond differently to the same roux. The first group (wine) turns into a wine sauce. The second group (milk) turns into a white sauce (béchamel sauce). The third group (tomato) turns into tomato sauce.[20] Although all resulting sauces may be equally delicious, the outcomes are unique even though the *identical treatment* (roux) was administered to each group. In other words, there is an interaction effect.

Interactions are not uncommon in studies of the effects of interventions and therefore should be examined

when possible to better understand who will benefit from a treatment. For example, the postural stability of children and adults may be different with the introduction of visual cues because children may be more dependent on such cues. Children may fall when they perceive their environment (walls) moving toward them, whereas adults may also use proprioceptive cues and not fall. The effect of coffee intake for children and adults also is different. Some children may tend to calm down, whereas adults become more stimulated.

Between-Subject versus Within-Subject Designs. Designs can also be classified according to whether (1) each subject is assigned to one group and only receives treatment given to that group (between-subject design) or (2) each subject receives all treatments (within-subject design). *Between-subject design* means that separate groups of people are formed and exposed to different treatments on the basis of group assignment. An example is an RCT. Outcomes from the different groups are then compared. This type of design is used when it is impossible or undesirable to expose persons to more than one level of the treatment (e.g., when one treatment effect can carry over to another, different teaching strategies, different surgical techniques).

Within-subject designs, also called *repeated measures designs* mean that every subject is exposed to all treatments and the outcomes for each subject are compared across these treatments (Figure 7-8). Although this may be a practical design in the clinic because each subject acts as his or her own control (compare treatment response with baseline response), a challenge in this kind of design is to manage sequence effects such as practice and fatigue.

True Experiments

True experiments offer the greatest control over threats to internal validity because they include a comparison group and randomly assign subjects into the groups. True exper-

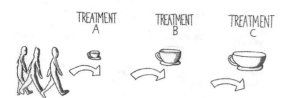

Figure 7-8. Within-subject design (also called *repeated measures design*) is useful when you want to expose the same individual to all treatments (e.g., different amounts of coffee).

iments are appropriate to determine efficacy of a therapeutic, educational, administrative intervention,[3] and are useful for evaluating interventions simultaneously or when carry-over effects of different treatments are likely.[12]

Randomized Clinical Trial.   The RCT (also a pretest–posttest control group design) is the classic example of an experimental design, and is used to determine the efficacy of a therapeutic intervention.[3,4] At least two groups (comparison groups) are involved—an experimental group and a control group. Subjects are randomly assigned to one of the two groups so that the characteristics of each group are homogeneous (similar) at the start of the study, as if they begin at the same starting line in a race. The experimental group undergoes the treatment, and the control group does not. The study is called *double blind* when neither the investigator nor the subjects know who is receiving the treatment. The results are analyzed to determine whether the experimental group has improved relative to the control group.[3] A slight variation of this design is indicated if it is unethical to withhold treatment, that is, to have a control group. In this case, a new treatment is compared with a conventional treatment.[12]

The advantage of RCTs is that they are less prone to bias and therefore provide some of the strongest medical evidence of causality. This design also is appropriate to control for carry-over effects among patients (i.e., whether lasting change is likely to occur) because the subjects typically receive one rather than multiple treatments. Some of the disadvantages of RCTs are expense, feasibility, such as trying to assign patients to a control group, and ethical issues, again such as whether or not to place patients in a control group.[11]

Posttest-Only Control Group Design.   This experimental design is similar to an RCT, but there is no pretest (no baseline measurement). It is indicated when baseline measure, the pretest, would affect the outcome of the study (called *reactivity*) or when a baseline measure is not possible. In other words, if administering a test will cue the patient on how to perform well later, the pretest becomes a confounder and should be avoided. This type of design improves the ability to generalize the results (external validity) because in life we usually do not

undergo pretests. Large sample sizes are recommended in this design to ensure similar group characteristics because you cannot verify homogeneity without the pretest.[4,12]

The Solomon Four-group Design.   This experimental design is a combination of the pretest-posttest and the posttest only control group designs, resulting in a four-group design. The advantages are improved internal and external validity. By studying the treatment effect on groups with and without a pretest, one can directly compare the reactive effects of testing between the groups. This design may be too expensive to implement. Nevertheless, it is included for completeness because it is fairly well known.[1,4]

Factorial Designs (Providing Multiple Treatments). Factorial design (true experiments and quasiexperiments) are used to examine the effect of more than one type of treatment (called a *factor*) on performance as discussed previously. The advantage of these designs is enhanced ability to generalize to the real world because studying the effect of only one treatment in isolation from other variables usually is artificial. Factorial designs allow the study of *interactions* such as the effect of a combination of treatments on performance or the effect of one treatment on two different groups (e.g., young and old).

Quasiexperimental Designs

It may be helpful to think of quasiexperimental designs as similar to experimental designs except that either a comparison group or the randomization process is absent. These designs therefore offer less control than do experimental designs over threats to the believability of a study.[12] Quasiexperimental and experimental designs are similar in that they involve manipulating an independent variable (treatment) rather than simply observing subjects in their natural setting.

Nonequivalent Pretest-Posttest Design.   This design is used when you have *intact (existing) groups* (e.g., two groups of patients with the same diagnosis, some of whom seek treatment and some of whom do not). Because you cannot randomly assign subjects into groups to ensure equivalence before the experiment begins, it is considered a quasiexperiment. Otherwise, it is similar to the classic pretest-posttest control group design described earlier. Intact groups, which may be importantly different in some characteristics, may respond differently over time (e.g., healing at different rates) or if baseline scores for the two groups are extremely different (called *regression to the mean*).[12] Thus internal validity can be compromised when groups are not equivalent in relevant characteristics at the beginning of the study.

Repeated Measures Designs.   As discussed above, in repeated measures designs (within-subject designs), every subject undergoes every treatment. There is no comparison group or random assignment into groups, but the treatment is manipulated. This kind of design offers a great deal of control because each person is compared with himself or herself. The design is useful to control for possible influence of individual variability (common among patients) because these differences are likely to remain constant.[12] Change can be attributed to the intervention. A second advantage of this design is that fewer subjects may be needed because the design is powerful (sensitive). Repeated measures designs are particularly useful for clinicians interested in how the same subjects or patients respond to different treatments.[12]

Because each subject receives each treatment, it is important that the order of treatments be systematically varied. This can be addressed through a counterbalanced or crossover design (the order is varied) so that the sequence of treatments does not become a confounding variable. That is, if tasks are always most difficult in the early trials, performance may be affected by this factor alone.

Repeated measures designs should not be implemented if the effects of one treatment carry over into the next treatment. That is, you cannot be sure which treatment was the effective one. If carry-over effects are anticipated, a between subjects design, described earlier, would be more appropriate.

Single-Case Experimental Designs (Time-Series Designs). The single-case experimental design is another example of a quasiexperimental design.[21] These designs are indicated when you want to examine trends, such as skill acquisition, over time in one subject or several subjects. The advantage of these designs are as follows: (1) skill acquisition and learning can be studied, (2) treatment effect can be dissociated from recovery rate, (3) individual response rather than average group response to treatment can be studied, (4) investigators know immediately rather than after statistical analysis whether performance is affected by treatment, (5) the design conforms to a clinical setting, and (6) there is no need to withhold treatment in multiple baseline designs.[12] A disadvantage of these designs is the problem of generalizing findings from one subject to a large population. This limitation can be addressed in part through replication. A controversial issue with single-case experimental designs is whether statistical analysis should be used.[21]

In general, multiple measures are taken until an established baseline trend is established. The investigator then administers treatment, and an outcome that is different from the projected trend is attributed to the treatment.

In *sequential introduction* and *withdrawal designs* (withdrawal designs, ABA designs), no change in performance is expected without treatment (phase A), a change is expected with treatment (phase B), and a return to baseline without treatment (phase A) establishes effectiveness of treatment. This design is indicated if withdrawing treatment is ethical and if no carry-over

(learning) effects preclude returning to baseline when treatment is withdrawn.

In *multiple-baseline designs*, several subjects or behaviors are studied at the same time. By staggering when treatment is introduced for each subject, the confounding effects of events (history) occurring during the study are controlled. These designs are particularly useful when you do not want to withhold treatment for ethical reasons or if the effects, such as learning, of the treatment are not reversible (when the effect will not reverse itself on withdrawal of the treatment).[12]

COMMON MISTAKES IN DESIGN

MISTAKE: NO MENTION OF A DESIGN

Students frequently fail to mention their design in their proposal, possibly because they are not certain what to call it. This is not entirely the students' fault because the same kind of research unfortunately can be described in numerous ways. For example, a correlational design also is considered a descriptive study, a preexperimental design, a cross-sectional design, or even a snapshot study. In each case, the researcher may be describing relationships at one point in time.

MISTAKE: MY DESIGN IS MY INSTRUMENT

Another mistake is confusing a design with an instrument. The design is the plan or blueprint of the study. On the other hand, the instrument is used simply to collect the data so that you can answer the question. For example, if you want to study the relationship between cigarette smoking and cancer, you may choose a correlational design because you are seeking to establish an association. The questionnaire used to collect the data is the instrument. In short, the design is not your instrument.

MISTAKE: CORRELATIONAL DESIGNS DEMONSTRATE CAUSE AND EFFECT

This is a big mistake. Students need to be careful not to use the terms *effect* and *cause* when they are really only capable of describing a relationship (an association or interdependence). Although this warning is in virtually every research textbook that ever filled a library shelf, the mistake still finds its way into research proposals. This flaw manifests itself when words such as *impact, influence, effectiveness, efficacy,* and *effect* improperly find their way into the conclusion section of a correlational design.

Example

If you go to a hospital, you will probably see a large number of sick people admitted. There may be a relationship or association between illness and hospitals.

They seem to go together. The larger the hospital, the more sick people there are. However, larger hospitals do not cause greater illness. Something else (disease or trauma) causes the illness that brings the patient to the available (larger) hospital.

Example

Rooster crowing and daybreak occur together. Although roosters may believe that they cause the sun to rise by crowing, the two are only related. Crowing does not cause the sun to rise.

REFERENCES

1. Nachmias CF, Nachmias D. *Research Methods in the Social Sciences.* 5th ed. New York: St. Martin's Press; 1996.
2. Bax M. Quantitative or qualitative research? [Editorial.] *Dev Med Child Neurol.* 1997;39:501.
3. Gehlbach SH. *Interpreting the Medical Literature.* 3rd ed. New York: McGraw-Hill; 1993.
4. Campbell DT, Stanley JC. *Experimental and Quasiexperimental Designs for Research.* Boston: Houghton Mifflin; 1963.
5. Wilkinson L. Task Force on Statistical Inference, APA Board of Scientific Affairs. Statistical methods in psychology journals: guidelines and explanations. *Am Psychol.* 1999;54:594–604.
6. Sackett DL, Wennberg JE. Choosing the best research design of each question: it's time to stop the squabbling over the "best" methods. *BMJ.* 1997;315:1636.
7. Tyler KL. A history of Parkinson's disease. In: Koller WC, ed. *Handbook of Parkinson's Disease.* New York: Marcel Dekker; 1992:1–13.
8. Hymes KB, Cheung T, Greene JB, et al. Kaposi's sarcoma in homosexual men: a report of eight cases. *Lancet.* 1981;2:598–600.
9. Bolger H. The case study method. In: Wolman BB, ed. *The Handbook of Clinical Psychology.* New York: McGraw-Hill; 1965:28–39.
10. Lashley KS. The accuracy of movement on the absence of excitation from the moving organ. *Am J Physiol.* 1917;43:169–194.
11. Peipert JF, Gifford DS, Boardman LA. Research design and methods of quantitative synthesis of medical evidence. *Obstet Gynecol.* 1997;90:473–478.
12. Portney LG, Watkins MP. *Foundations of Clinical Research: Applications to Practice.* Upper Saddle River, N.J.: Prentice Hall; 2000.
13. Piaget J. *The Child's Construction of Reality.* London: Routledge & Kegan Paul; 1955.
14. McGraw MB. *Growth: a Study of Johnny and Jimmy.* New York: Appleton-Century; 1935.
15. Hamill PV, Drizd TA, Johnson CL, et al. Physical growth: National Center for Health Statistics percentiles. *Am J Clin Nutr.* 1979;32:607–629.
16. Batavia AI. Of wheelchairs and managed care. *Health Aff (Millwood).* 1999;18:177–182.
17. Morse JM, Field PA. *Qualitative Research Methods for Health Professionals.* 2nd ed. Thousand Oaks, Calif: Sage Publications; 1995.
18. Reswick JB. What constitutes valid research? Qualitative vs. quantitative research. *J Rehabil Res Dev.* 1994;31:vii–ix.
19. Greenhalgh T, Taylor R. How to read a paper: papers that go beyond numbers (qualitative research). *BMJ.* 1997;315:740–743.
20. Gisslen W. *Professional Cooking.* 2nd ed. New York: John Wiley & Sons; 1989.
21. Hersen M, Barlow DH. *Single Case Experimental Designs: Strategies for Studying Behavior Change.* Oxford, England: Pergamon Press; 1982.

8
Sampling

STUDYING PEOPLE

Once you have identified a question, you will need a group of persons to study. Although it would be fine to study every person in the world who may help answer your question (the population), this is rarely done in practice.[1]

A WORD ABOUT POPULATIONS

When we talk about populations in research, we typically mean a very large group of persons, animals, events, places, or things that share a characteristic.[1] The persons, places, or things identified as the population may not all be available to the researcher. They provide only the potential for observation; only some of these persons, places, or things probably will be studied.[2] Examples include all young men in New York City who have HIV infection. Another population could be all young men in the United States who have HIV infection.

THE PROBLEM: TOO MANY PEOPLE

It would be difficult if not impossible to include the entire population of interest in your study. First, you would have to locate every one of them (could be millions or at least thousands of people). Next you would have to contact and arrange for every one of them to participate in the study. This would be a logistical and financial nightmare because you would have to contact them, perhaps arrange for transportation, and provide some compensation for travel. Whereas inviting, scheduling, and compensating 30 or even a couple hundred people in your study would be possible, studying hundreds of thousands if not millions of people (the entire population) would not be.

THE SOLUTION: SAMPLE IT

The solution is to sample a small segment of the population you are interested in studying. The trick is to choose a sample that represents the larger population. In other words, you want the sample to be a miniature version of the population so that it is similar in character but manageable in size. It is crucial to understand that who is studied (the population) will determine how the study is interpreted.[2] Simply put, you cannot learn about physician practice patterns if you include nurses and physician assistants in the study.

TWO BASIC WAYS TO SAMPLE

The two major ways to sample a population are by probabilistic sampling and nonprobabilistic sampling.

PROBABILISTIC SAMPLING

Researchers deal with the problem of studying a large population simply by studying a smaller portion of the entire segment of society and assuming that the smaller portion is representative of the larger group they want to know about. This is called *probabilistic sampling* because selection of the sample is left to chance.[3,4] First identify the entire segment of society (target population) you want to study. Then randomly select a small portion of that population. The key to the word *random* is that every person in the population has an *equal chance* of being selected for the study. The following example is used to describe four methods of probabilistic sampling—simple random sampling, systematic sampling, stratified sampling, and cluster sampling. Each method has advantages.

Example: The Taste Tester

It is the year 1200, and you have the dubious honor of being the food taster for the King of England. Your job is to taste appetizers for a party to make sure the king and the rest of the royal family are not poisoned. Of course, if you are good at your job, you'll eat the food and die so that the king and his family will not.

The problem is that there are 500 rooms in the castle and there is food in every one. It would be impossible for you to taste all 10,000 appetizers in the castle, and for obvious reasons, you cannot get anyone to help you with your task. Furthermore, if you were to eat them all, what would the royal family and their guests eat?

The solution is to sample a few of the entire number of appetizers randomly. Random sampling is the best method of acquiring a representative segment of the population short of sampling the entire population of appetizers. If you do not find any poisonous appetizers in the small, randomly selected sample, you can assume that there are also no poisonous appetizers on the trays distributed throughout the castle. Of course, there is always a chance that you missed a poisonous appetizer, and then you are out of a job, if not executed.

Simple Random Selection

One way to sample the entire supply of appetizers is simple random selection.[3,4] You find every appetizer in the castle and assign it a number. If there are 10,000 appetizers, you number them from 1 to 10,000. You then write each number on an identical piece of paper, place all the numbers (the entire population) in a container, close your eyes, and pick a sample, for example, 300 pieces of paper, randomly from the hat so that each appetizer has an equal chance of being picked. You then eat only the appetizers that correspond to the numbers selected at randomly from the hat.

A similar way to select the smaller sample is to use an existing table of random numbers (found in most research books) and simply go down or across the table, line by line, until the first 300 numbers that correspond to the 10,000 appetizers are identified. Technically, using a table of random numbers or a computer-generated program is preferred to a physical mechanism such as a picking from a hat or drum because mechanical methods can be corrupted by nonrandom picks, as in the Vietnam draft lottery, if the drum is not turned sufficiently.[2]

Systematic Sampling

Although simple random selection may be useful for a small population, 10,000 is too many to number unless they are already numbered for some reason. For large populations, it may be easier simply to select one appetizer at random and then systematically skip a given number, for example 33, before selecting another appetizer.[3,4] You go from room to room and eat one appetizer, skip the next 33 you see, and then eat the next one until you either select or skip all 10,000 appetizers throughout the castle. Why 33? If I have 10,000 appetizers and skip every 33, I should be able to cover practically the entire castle (all 10,000 appetizers) while I select only 300 to eat (10,000/300 = 33).

Stratified Sampling

If you know the proportion of the king's favorite appetizers (e.g., 40% of the 10,000, or 4000 appetizers), the proportion of the queen's favorite appetizers (30% of 10,000, or 3000 appetizers), and the proportion of the prince's favorite appetizers (30% of 10,000, or 3000 appetizers), you can sample the population in these proportions (proportional stratified sample). Doing so helps ensure that a representative proportion of each favorite kind of appetizer is sampled. In other words, you are randomly selecting from three subgroups (each stratum), the favorites.[3,4]

You can identify the king's favorites in the castle and randomly select 40% of the total size of your sample (40% of 300 = 120 appetizers). You then identify the queen's favorites in the castle and randomly select another 30% of the total sample size (30% of 300 = 90 appetizers). Finally, you identify the prince's favorites and randomly select the final 30% of your total sample size (30% of 300 = 90 appetizers). The total sample (120 + 90 + 90 = 300 appetizers) then reflects the proportion of favorite appetizers in the population (4000 + 3000 + 3000) throughout the castle.

Cluster Sampling

Another way to randomly select your sample from an *extremely large population* is to identify clusters of populations first and then randomly select the sample from each cluster.[3,4] Because you have a large population of appetizers (10,000) and 500 rooms (500 clusters) where you can find this population, you can first randomly select 30 rooms of the 500 and from each of the 30 rooms randomly select 10 appetizers to obtain a representative sample.

NONPROBABILISTIC SAMPLING: THE COLD HARD TRUTH

The cold hard truth is that although probabilistic sampling such as random sampling is common in research involving questionnaires, it is rare in clinical research in which you are conducting experiments. Instead many researchers use nonprobabilistic sampling because it is easier and more practical than probabilistic sampling and sometimes is the only way to reach a particular population. It involves choosing the sample in a manner in which not all subjects in the population of interest have an equal chance of being selected. Using this method, you are more likely to miss the poisonous appetizer in the example. Because researchers do not study samples that are representative of the larger population, they must limit their conclusions about the findings to the defined group characteristics of the subjects in the study.[5] Four methods of nonprobabilistic sampling will be discussed—convenience, snowball, quota, and purposeful sampling.

Convenience Sampling: Availability

In convenience sampling, the investigator simply finds anyone who fits the criteria for the study.[3,4] Subjects are easy or convenient to recruit.[5] Investigators typically place advertisements in newspapers and post flyers with the specific criteria needed. "If you're a person who has had a right cerebral vascular accident and are between the ages of 40 and 77 years and walks, that's what we're looking for. You're in the study. When are you available?" It is a sample of convenience for the researcher.

Snowball Sampling: Word of Mouth

Snowball sampling is similar to convenience sample except that you ask those who have just participated in the study to find friends or similar patients who also may be interested in being subjects in the study.[3,4] This is a useful approach if it is difficult to locate the population for your study. If you have just evaluated a subject who has had a stroke, he or she may attend a stroke support group and make an announcement about the study to other group members. Snowball sampling has the advantage of word of mouth advertising for difficult to locate populations.

Quota Sampling: Proportions

Quota sampling selects people from the population on the basis of known proportions in the population. If, for example, you want to survey physical therapists in the United States, and sex may influence responses, you may want to select men and women according to their proportions in the profession (e.g., x% men, y% women). The problem is that because every person in the population does not have an equal chance of being selected (nonprobabilistic sampling), the resulting sample may not accurately reflect the opinions of the population.

Purposeful Sampling: Hand-picked

When the investigator is specifically searching for subjects or patients with certain criteria to meet the needs of a study, it is called *purposeful sampling*. The criteria may be to include typical patients or patients with a given disease or history. Invitation is up to the judgment of the investigator.

SUMMARY

Although probabilistic sampling such as random sampling allows investigators to infer findings from their sample to the population, the same cannot be said for nonprobabilistic sampling such as convenience sampling. Inferences made from nonrepresentative samples, such as convenience sampling, should be interpreted with caution. Clearly defined samples that are nonrandomly selected require clinical judgment to assess the degree of ability to generalize the findings to a population.[6] The representativeness of a convenience sample may be strengthened, at times, by including a wide range of well-defined characteristics found among the identified population.[2]

THINGS TO DO

1. Review three research reports and determine the type of sampling mentioned in the study (note that convenience sampling is common in medical reports). Was the sampling method appropriate for the type of study?
2. Identify a patient population in the literature. Describe how you would sample this population using the eight sampling designs (methods) described in this chapter. Which sampling design would be most appropriate for your study?

REFERENCES

1. Greenfield MLVH, Kuhn JE, Wojtys EM. A statistics primer. *Am J Sports Med.* 1996;24:393–395.
2. Wilkinson L. Task Force on Statistical Inference, APA Board of Scientific Affairs. Statistical methods in psychology journals: guidelines and explanations. *Am Psychol.* 1999;54:594–604.
3. Portney LG, Watkins MP. *Foundations of Clinical Research: Applications to Practice.* Upper Saddle River, N.J.: Prentice Hall; 2000.
4. Nachmias CF, Nachmias D. *Research Methods in the Social Sciences.* 5th ed. New York: St. Martin's Press; 1996.
5. Light RJ, Singer JD, Willett JB. *By Design: Planning Research on Higher Education.* Cambridge, Mass: Harvard University Press; 1990.
6. Munro BH, Page EB. *Statistical Methods for Health Care Research.* 2nd ed. Philadelphia: JB Lippincott; 1993.

9

Measurement

One of the investigator's goals is to try to find a measuring instrument that will answer a question in a believable way. The more accurate and consistent your measurements are, the more believable your answer will be.

MEASUREMENT INSTRUMENTS AND SCIENCE

Advancement of knowledge in science often awaits improvements in measurement techniques. Examples can be found in many fields.[1]

THE GAITS OF HORSES

In the 1800s, there was a controversy about whether at any phase of a horse's trot all four feet are off the ground. Muybridge[2] developed a method of taking pictures clear enough to demonstrate for the first time that all four hooves can leave the ground simultaneously during a trot.

THE MILKY WAY

In the 1600s, the image over the sky was called the Milky Way because it appeared milky. Galileo developed a telescope and observed that the milky vision was actually made up of individual stars.[3]

ELECTRICAL NERVE IMPULSES

Galen's view that the nervous system was hollow and acted as a gland to carry the vital spirits was taught until the 1700s. Galvani suggested the notion of electrical nerve impulses in the 1700s but was not able to confirm his idea until Emil Du Bois-Reymond developed an instrument to measure the phenomenon.[4,5]

THE NERVE DOCTRINE AND SYNAPSE

In 1663, Robert Hooke, using an instrument with two lenses called a *compound microscope,* saw small holes in cork slices. He called these holes *cells.*[6] In 1837, Purkinje gave the first detailed account of nerve cells he examined with an improved microscope. The cell was described as having a main body and a tail.[5] Using a stain to improve contrast, Golgi was able to describe dendrites, but the junction, which was thought by many to be continuous, was not clear. In 1889, Cajal improved the Golgi stain and was able to clearly observe each nerve cell as separate rather than continuous (the neuron doctrine). In 1931, investigators using an electron microscope observed synapses (gap between nerve cells) at 20,000 times their actual size.

THEORY OF MUSCLE CONTRACTION

Two filament theories were developed in attempts to explain the contraction of muscle. The continuous filament theory suggests that actin and myosin (the contractile proteins) combine into one continuous filament that folds to shorten (i.e., contract). Observations with an electron microscope, however, support an alternative sliding filament theory of muscle contraction. Proteins slide rather than fold during muscle contraction.[7]

THE PERFECT MEASURING INSTRUMENT DOES NOT EXIST

Although there is a strong tendency to use the best instrument for a study, the reality is that *no perfect instrument exists.* Every instrument has strengths and weaknesses, and there is some measurement error inherent in all instruments. Even if you were to come close to perfection, the measurement still may not be appropriate for your study. The key is to choose an instrument that can help answer your research question.

THE GIGO LAW: GARBAGE IN, GARBAGE OUT

No matter how good or expensive your measuring instrument is, if you do not know how to use it or if you do not apply standardized procedures to your subjects while you collect data with the instrument, your data will be meaningless. In other words, if your procedures (methods) are sloppy, your data will obey the GIGO law: garbage in, garbage out (Figure 9-1).

THE UNCERTAINTY OF MEASUREMENT

It may be surprising or even shocking to realize that when we measure anything, we cannot be sure that the measurement is correct.[8] In fact, if you measure anything carefully 100 times with a continuous measure (e.g., one person's height with a tape measure), you are bound to record many slightly different measurements. How then can you be sure what a person's true height is? The scientific way is to take an average of all 100 (or however many) measurements you record.[9] The average is a summary value that tells you the number on which all the scores center.

SIGNAL AND NOISE

The average is the best estimate of a score and can be considered the signal or important information concerning a measurement (height in this example). The measurements you take that vary around the average score reflect the variability, scatter, or spread of the score. The variability can be viewed as "noise" in the measurement.[10]

ALL SCORES ARE A COMBINATION OF A TRUE VALUE AND MEASUREMENT ERROR

Every measurement you take in life is actually a combination of the true value (signal) and measurement error (noise).[11,12] Factors that contribute to measurement error (and screw up your data) include (1) measuring mistakes made by the investigator, (2) day-to-day changes in the subjects, (3) inferior measuring instruments, or (4) changes in the environment (e.g., temperature and humidity can affect electronic instruments).

The more careful you are at reducing measurement error in your study, the closer the measures will be to the true value (signal), and the less variable (noise) your measurements will be. If you are careless taking measurements or if your measuring instrument is inferior, there will be greater variability (noise) in your measurements and therefore greater difficulty in recording the true value (Figure 9-2).

Even the act of measuring something can sometimes alter the measurement. A common example is the change in a person's gait or posture when the individual is aware of being observed. In quantum physics, the act of measuring an electron changes its behavior because the measurement involves a disruptive interaction with the electron.[13] Measuring something is not as easy as it seems.

HOW GOOD IS YOUR MEASURING INSTRUMENT?

The quality of a measuring instrument is determined by means of evaluating its validity (accuracy) and reliability

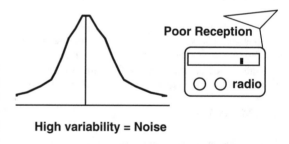

Poor Reception

High variability = Noise

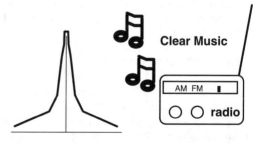

Clear Music

Low variability = Signal (information)

Figure 9-2.   Variability in data is analogous to listening to a radio station with a broken antenna. You cannot hear the music (information) because there is too much background static (noise).

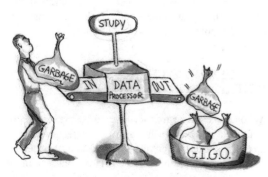

Figure 9-1.   If you do not understand the limits of your measuring instrument, your data may be meaningless. The law of GIGO means garbage in, garbage out.

(consistency). The methods section of a report should include information about the validity and reliability of the instruments. The only way to know whether the instrument possesses validity and reliability for a particular population is if these values are reported or you evaluate it (see Chapter 23). Validity and reliability are commonly assessed with a correlation coefficient (an index) that ranges from 0 to 1—the higher the absolute value, the stronger is the measure. For acceptable validity of clinical measures, a correlation of 0.90 or higher is desirable.[12]

VALIDITY

Validity (truthfulness) is extremely important in a measuring instrument. It implies that the instrument measures accurately what it purports to measure. There are several types of validity—face, content, criteria, concurrent, predictive, and construct.[12,14]

Face Validity

If an instrument has face, or apparent, validity, *it looks or appears* to be relevant for that particular measurement. Face validity is a subjective assessment[14] and is a very low standard of validity but is better than nothing (barely). Face validity can be important, however, because the investigator and subject need to be convinced that the instrument appears to measure what it purports to measure. Subjects may be less interested in participating in research if measures do not appear relevant. If you show someone a goniometer and state that it is used to measure weight loss, that person would be correct in saying the instrument lacks face validity.[12]

Content Validity

If an instrument, such as a test, has content validity, it contains a representative sample of questions on a subject matter. If you write an anatomy exam and some of the questions have to do with soap operas rather than muscles, bones, and organs, you can say the test lacks content validity. Content validity can be determined by a panel of experts (authorities) on the subject matter and is one element of validation of questionnaires.[12]

Criterion Validity

If an instrument has criterion validity, the measurements obtained are comparable with those obtained with an existing, well-accepted instrument (Figure 9-3). If the well-accepted instrument and your instrument are compared with each other at the same time, *concurrent validity* is being tested. Ideally, you want to compare your instrument with the most-accepted instrument for a particular measurement (also called the *standard of reference* or *gold standard*). For example, although the goniometer is well-accepted for measuring joint angles, a radiograph is the standard of reference because one can measure the actual joint articulation with less error on film rather than over skin and muscle.

Predictive Validity

If an instrument is purported to allow predictions about an outcome, it is said to possess predictive validity. A classic example in education is the validity of SAT scores in predicting grade point averages in college. In medicine and physical rehabilitation, instruments that enable investigators to accurately predict the number of days until

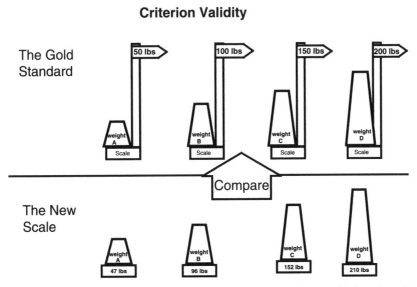

Figure 9-3. Criterion validity is used to compare the accuracy of a new instrument with that of a well-accepted instrument.

recovery on the basis of initial evaluation scores would be said to have predictive validity.

Construct Validity

If an instrument has construct validity, it can measure an abstract concept or construct (these are things you usually cannot touch physically). In education, for example, intelligence is a construct measured on several dimensions with intelligence tests. In psychology, a measure of ability to adjust to a physical disability may possess construct validity if expected associations with other characteristics such as attitude about the future and sense of self-worth can be demonstrated.[15] In medicine and physical rehabilitation, constructs such as pain, which is not a concrete phenomenon or directly observable, require validity measures for adequate evaluation of the efficacy of treatment.[12] Because measures such as pain have several dimensions, more than one instrument may be needed to capture the multidimensional nature of its construct.[12]

RELIABILITY

Reliability refers to the ability of an instrument to repeatedly measure the same phenomenon.[12] In general, when we examine the similarity of measurements, we assess their agreement (Figure 9-4) (see Chapters 12 and 22). When we examine how well measures correspond (e.g., scores vary up and down together), we are assessing *consistency of ranking* (see Chapter 12).

Test-Retest Reliability

Test-retest reliability answers the question "How repeatable (or stable) is the instrument at taking measurements?" It refers to the instrument's ability of measuring something on two separate occasions—a test and a retest. Typically you evaluate reliability over the range of values the instrument is capable of measuring.

Test-retest reliability is crucial because you want to know the instrument is dependable. If your instrument lacks test-retest reliability, you cannot be certain whether changes in your patient are caused by a treatment or by the mercurial nature of your measuring instrument.

Rater Reliability

Rater reliability answers the question, "Do persons taking the measurements with the instrument obtain consistent results?"

Intrarater Reliability.   Intrarater reliability refers to the ability of an investigator who takes measurements to obtain the same result on more than one occasion (Figure 9-5). This form of reliability is crucial because one needs to know whether one investigator's (rater's) procedure of measurement is dependable. This can be an important form of reliability because most instruments necessitate that the investigator prepare the subject in an appropriate manner for the experiment. If the investigator is not consistent in preparing the subject or in operating the equipment, the measurements may be inconsistent simply because of inconsistent use of the instruments (see Chapter 18).

Interrater Reliability.   Interrater reliability refers to the ability of two or more different investigators (raters) to measure the same thing. This form of reliability is crucial if more than one investigator is involved in measuring subjects in the same study. If two investigators' measurements lack correspondence, measurements taken during the study may be inconsistent simply because of variations in how two investigators use the same equipment (Figure 9-6) (see Chapter 18).

Test-Retest Reliability

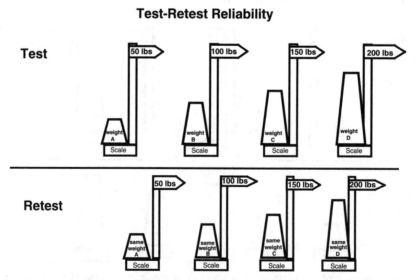

Figure 9-4.   Test-retest reliability measures possess good agreement if an instrument produces similar or identical scores on separate occasions.

Intrarater Reliability

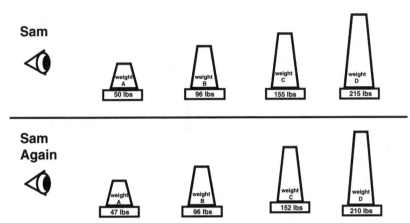

Figure 9-5.   Intrarater reliability reflects the stability of one person's data collection procedures at separate points in time. In this example, Sam's measurements are assessed twice and are similar.

Interrater Reliability

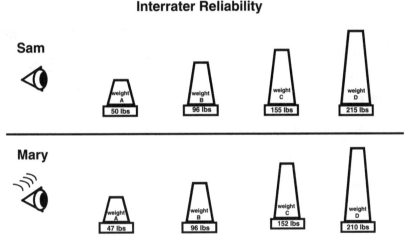

Figure 9-6.   Interrater reliability is important if two or more investigators are collecting data. In this example, Sam's and Mary's measurements of the same phenomena are similar.

Reliability (Internal Consistency) of Pencil and Paper Tests

This type of reliability answers the question, "Do the questions (items) on a test all measure the same trait or characteristic?"

Split-half Reliability.   Split-half reliability evaluates the consistency of two parts of the same measuring instrument and is commonly used to establish the internal consistency of questionnaires. For example, if you had only one questionnaire, you might split it into two parts (e.g., even-numbered and odd-numbered questions) to determine whether subjects respond in a consistent manner to both halves of the questionnaire.[12]

Test Item Reliability.   Test item reliability is used to evaluate how each question (item) relates to the other questions (items) in an instrument.

Summary

The validity and reliability of measurements are crucial to believing a study. In most instances not all types of validity and reliability are reported in one study. Rather, information deemed appropriate in the particular study is reported. For example, split-half reliability is not reported if a pencil and paper test is not administered in the study. On the other hand, if more than one investigator is rating performance, interrater reliability for the population under study should be reported.

CHARACTERISTICS OF ELECTRONIC MEASURING INSTRUMENTS

Electronic instrumentation and sensors often are evaluated by the manufacturers and can provide useful information about the measuring characteristics of a device.

This information can help investigators determine whether the instrument is appropriate to measure the phenomena in their studies. Because other researchers may want to replicate the study with the same instruments, it is important that model numbers and manufacturer addresses be included in a research report. Some measurement characteristics include accuracy, precision, range, threshold, sensitivity, and sampling rates.

Accuracy

The accuracy of a sensor is a measure of the difference between the output and the actual value.[11] The absolute difference is called the absolute error.[8] If you weigh 100 pounds (45 kg) (true value), and your scale reads 104 or 96 pounds (47 or 43 kg) when you stand on it, your scale has an absolute error of 4 pounds (2 kg).

The constant error is a signed difference (degree of overshooting or undershooting) rather than the absolute difference. If you weigh 100 pounds (true value) and your scale measures 104 pounds when you stand on it, your scale has a positive constant error of +4 pounds (Figure 9-7). If you weigh 100 pounds and your scale measures 96 pounds when you stand on it, your scale has a negative constant error of −4 pounds (Figure 9-8).

Precision

Precision refers to the reproducibility or repeatability of the same measurement. If an instrument has precision, it measures the same value exactly each time.[8,11] If you weigh 100 pounds and your scale measures 100 pounds each time you stand on it, your scale is precise. An instrument's measurements can be highly reproducible but inaccurate. In fact, measurements can be accurate and precise, accurate but imprecise, inaccurate but precise, or inaccurate and imprecise (Figures 9-9 through 9-12).

The Uncertainty of a Scale: Significant Figures

The smaller the interval that can be confidently read from the scale of an instrument, the more precise is the measurement.[8] For example, some goniometers show intervals that are 1 degree apart whereas others have scales with intervals that are 5 degrees apart.

Constant Error: Overshooting

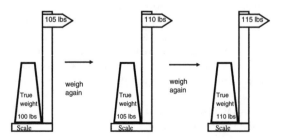

Figure 9-7. Positive constant error or overshooting occurs when the output of a measuring instrument is higher than the true value.

Constant Error: Undershooting

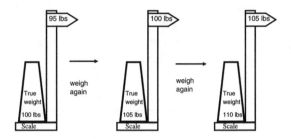

Figure 9-8. Negative constant error or undershooting occurs when the output of a measuring instrument is lower than the true value.

Precise & Accurate

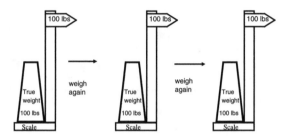

Figure 9-9. An instrument is both accurate and precise when it measures the true value consistently.

Imprecise but Accurate (on average)

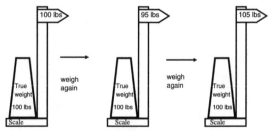

Figure 9-10. An instrument is accurate but imprecise when it measures a correct value (on average) but individual scores vary. In this example, the average of all scores equals the "true" weight of 100 pounds, but each individual score is not 100 pounds.

Precise but Inaccurate

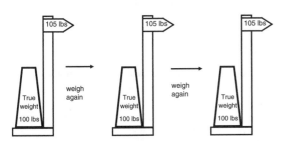

Figure 9-11. An instrument is inaccurate but precise when it measures an incorrect value consistently.

Imprecise & Inaccurate

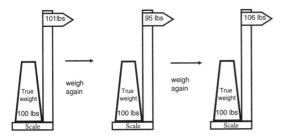

Figure 9-12. An instrument is both inaccurate and imprecise when it does not measure the true value accurately or consistently. In other words, it is useless.

Range

The range of an instrument refers to the full scope of measurements that can be recorded with the instrument.[11] A sphygmomanometer has a readable measuring range from 0 mm Hg to 300 mm Hg. If you are measuring pressure above this level, you need to use a different instrument.

A goniometer that measures up to 180 degrees may not have sufficient range for measuring the hip range of dancers. This is because dancers may exhibit a greater range of hip mobility than the goniometer is capable of recording. In this case, a universal (360-degree) goniometer would be appropriate.

If you weigh 200 pounds (90 kg) and your scale only has a range from 0 to 180 pounds (81 kg), you need a scale with a wider range (at least up to 200 pounds and perhaps 10% more as an engineering rule of thumb, that is 220 pounds [99 kg]; C. Mason, M.S.B.E., oral communication, May 23, 2000). Exceeding the range of a device is called the *ceiling effect*. That is, the instrument cannot measure anything higher than the high-end point of the scale. If the range of a scale is 25 to 100 pounds (11 to 45 kg) and you weigh less than 25 pounds, the scale will not be capable of measuring the true value. In this case, the problem is called a *floor effect* because the device cannot measure lower values (Figure 9-13).

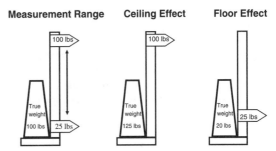

Figure 9-13. Ceiling effects occur when the true value (e.g., 125 pounds [56 kg]) exceeds the measurement range of the instrument (e.g., exceeds 100 pounds [45 kg]). Floor effects occur when the true value (e.g., 20 pounds [9 kg]) is below the measurement range of the instrument (e.g., 25 pounds [11 kg]) so that no recorded value is registered.

Threshold

The *threshold* is the lowest level of input that the measuring instrument can record. When you are measuring an activity such as walking on a mat that electronically records footprints with conductive ink, you want to know the minimum weight the mat can record. If the threshold of a sensor is 40 pounds (18 kg), the activity of young subjects (those who weigh less than 40 pounds) will not be recorded.[11]

Sensitivity

The *sensitivity* of a sensor refers to the smallest input that will register a detectable change in the output.[11] Insensitive measuring instruments may not sufficiently detect small changes in phenomena.

Sampling Rate

Sampling rate refers to the ability of a measuring instrument to record an activity a specified number of times within a time period, usually in Hertz (cycles/second or frames/second). If you are measuring portions of a performance over time, such as walking, then you need to be concerned about the sampling rate of the instrument. Sampling rate is important to consider when recording movement (filming), forces (force plate), and electromyographic activity because you do not want to miss a crucial aspect of the performance.

The sampling rate needed for a study depends on the activity being recorded. The faster the activity, the higher the sampling rate has to be. Recording running requires a higher sampling rate than recording walking. For example, if a video camera samples a burglary in a 24-hour delicatessen every 5 seconds (12 per minute), it will probably capture the crime on film. If, however, the camera samples the burglary only once every minute (1 per minute), the crime may not appear on videotape if the crook is quick enough (less than 1 minute and between samples).

THE INFORMATION IN A SCORE: LEVELS OF MEASUREMENT

Every instrument provides a specific amount of information in a measurement (*level of measurement*) that may or may not be appropriate to answer your question. There are four levels of measurement—nominal (or categorical), ordinal, interval, and ratio.[12,14] The higher the level of measurement, the greater the information in a score. A higher measurement level (above nominal level) also may offer greater choices for analyzing data. In general, it is desirable to use a higher level of measurement (interval, ratio) because it improves the power (sensitivity) of your study.

Nominal Level

Nominal data, the lowest level of measurement, are used to measure how many subjects fit into a particular category, such as religion (Catholic, Jewish, Buddhist, Islamic), sex (male, female), blood pressure (normal, hypertensive), pain (yes, no), or level of function (independent, dependent). Nominal data are often collected with demographic questionnaires and surveys.

Ordinal Level

Ordinal measures are frequently collected in questionnaires and surveys. They provide additional information about the relative order or rank of a score. A common example is horse racing, in which a horse can win (finish first), show (finish second), or place (finish third). Other examples of ordinal measures include blood pressure (low, normal, high), attitudes (strongly disagree, disagree, neutral, agree, strongly agree), level of function (dependent, maximal assist, moderate assist, minimal assist, independent), and strength (zero, trace, poor, fair, good, normal). Many clinical measures in physical rehabilitation are ordinal in nature. The differences between levels or grades on an ordinal scale are not necessarily equal. Hence, trace strength (a twitch) may be only slightly greater than zero (no muscle activity), and poor strength (causing joint movement) may be substantially greater than muscle twitch strength.

Interval and Ratio Level

Interval and ratio data provide more precise information than do ordinal data. As with ordinal measures, the scores are ordered or ranked. The differences between measurement divisions are equally spaced for both interval and ratio data, which makes interpretation of subject performance less ambiguous and scores more amenable to math operations. An example of an interval measure is the Fahrenheit scale, on which degrees are equally spaced but there is no zero

(baseline) point. Examples of ratio measures include joint angle (degrees), force (pounds), and pressure (mm Hg) in which intervals are equally spaced and there is a baseline point (e.g., 0 degrees; 0 pounds, 0 mm Hg).

Summary

It is generally to your advantage to choose an instrument with which you can collect as much information about a score as possible if that information is necessary to answer your question. Choosing such an instrument increases the power or sensitivity of your method.[10] For example, pain can be measured at a nominal level (no pain, pain) or ordinal level (no pain, little pain, some pain, great deal of pain, unbearable) with a questionnaire as the instrument. Additional information about pain can be measured at a ratio level with an instrument that has a visual analog scale. The subject is asked, "How much pain do you experience on this 100 mm line?" The subject can indicate 0 mm, 50 mm, 100 mm, or anywhere in between.

EXAMPLES

The following are examples of levels of measurement for different clinical outcomes (performances, scores, dependent variables).

Pain
1. Nominal level (Instrument: questionnaire)
   Type of Question: Do you have pain?
   Yes   No
2. Ordinal level (Instrument: questionnaire)
   Type of Question: What level of pain do you experience?
   A lot   Some   None
3. Ratio level (Instrument: visual analog scale)
   Type of Question: How much pain do you experience on a 0 mm to 100 mm scale?
   100 mm   3 mm   2 mm   1 mm   0 mm

Joint Range of Motion
1. Nominal level (visual inspection)
   Type of Question: Is joint motion limited?
   No (within normal limits)   Yes
2. Ordinal level (visual inspection)
   Type of Question: How limited is joint motion?
   Ankylosed   Maximal limitation
   Moderate limitation   Mild limitation
   No limitations   Hypermobile
3. Ratio level (degrees of joint motion; Instrument: goniometer)
   Type of Question: How many degrees of motion are available?
   180 degrees   15 degrees   10 degrees
   5 degrees   0 degrees

Strength

1. Nominal level (gross examination)
   Type of Question: Is strength normal?
   Within normal limits   Not within normal limits
2. Ordinal level (Instrument: manual muscle test)
   Type of Question: What is the grade of strength?
   Normal   Good   Fair   Poor   Trace   Zero
3. Ratio level (Instrument: dynamometer)
   Type of Question: How many pounds of force can
   the subject exert?
   90 lb   1.1 lb   0 lb

Posture

1. Nominal level (inspection)
   Type of Question: What kind of posture is present?
   Ideal   Scoliosis   Kyphosis
   Are there postural deviations?
   Yes   No
2. Ordinal level (inspection)
   Type of Question: How much deformity is present?
   Severe   Moderate   Mild   None
3. Ratio level (Instrument: centimeters from plumb line)
   Type of Question: How much postural deviation is
   present?
   5 cm   1 cm   0 cm

Gait

1. Nominal level (visual inspection)
   Type of Question: Can the person walk?
   Yes (ambulatory)   No (nonambulatory)
2. Ordinal level (gross gait evaluation)
   Type of Question: How much help does the person
   need to walk?
   Total assistance (nonambulatory)
   Maximal assistance   Moderate assistance
   Minimal assistance   Verbal cueing   Independent
3. Ratio level (Instruments: videotape, stopwatch, tape
   measure)
   Type of Question: How fast can the person walk?
   1.0 m/s   0.25 m/s   0 m/s

THINGS TO DO

1. Identify three outcome measures in your field (e.g.,
   gait, reflexes, anxiety, depression, self-concept) and
   list all instruments that have been developed to measure this outcome. Next to each outcome, record the
   level of measurement of the instrument.

2. Choose a measuring instrument in your field. Describe
   all the types of validity that can be assessed for this
   instrument. What important information does each
   form of validity provide?
3. Choose another measuring instrument in your field.
   Describe all the types of reliability that can be
   assessed for this instrument. What important information does each form of reliability provide?

REFERENCES

1. Rensberger B. *How the World Works: A Guide to Science's Greatest Discoveries.* New York: Quill, William,
   Morrow; 1986.
2. Muybridge E. *Animals in Motion.* LS Brown, ed. New
   York: Dover; 1957.
3. Hart MH. *The 100: A Ranking of the Most Influential
   Persons in History.* Secaucus, N.J.: Citadel Press; 1987.
4. Jeannerod M. *The Brain Machine: The Development of
   Neurophysiological Thought.* Cambridge, Mass: Harvard University Press; 1985.
5. McGrew RE. *Encyclopedia of Medical History.* New
   York: McGraw-Hill; 1985.
6. Hawkes N. *Early Scientific Instruments.* New York:
   Abbeville Press; 1981.
7. West JR, ed. *Best and Taylor's Physiological Basis of
   Medical Practice.* 12th ed. Baltimore: Williams &
   Wilkins; 1991.
8. Kruglak H, Moore JT. *Schaum's Outline of Theory and
   Problems of Basic Mathematics with Application to Science and Technology.* New York: McGraw-Hill; 1973.
9. Feinstein AR. On exorcizing the ghost of Gauss and the
   curse of Kelvin. *MD Comput.*1992;9:303–323.
10. Light RJ, Singer JD, Willett JB. *By Design: Planning
    Research on Higher Education.* Cambridge, Mass:
    Harvard University Press; 1990.
11. Carr JJ. *Sensors and Circuits: Sensors, Transducers,
    and Supporting Circuits for Electronic Instrumenta-
    tions, Measurement, and Control.* Englewood Cliffs,
    N.J.: PTR Prentice Hall; 1993.
12. Portney LG, Watkins MP. *Foundations of Clinical
    Research: Applications to Practice.* Upper Saddle
    River, N.J.: Prentice Hall; 2000.
13. Hazen RM, Trefil J. *Science Matters: Achieving Scien-
    tific Literacy.* New York: Doubleday; 1991.
14. Nachmias CF, Nachmias D. *Research Methods in the
    Social Sciences.* 5th ed. New York: St. Martin's Press;
    1996.
15. Sim J, Arnell P. Measurement validity in physical ther-
    apy research. *Phys Ther.* 1993;73:102–109.

10

Descriptive Statistics

STATISTICS: A NUMERICAL SUMMARY

A statistic is a numerical summary. There are two kinds of statistics—descriptive and inferential. Descriptive statistics are used to describe the actual subjects encountered in a study. They are necessary for all research, whether the study is essentially descriptive in nature or part of a hypothesis testing (inferential) design. Inferential statistics are used to generalize findings from a study to the larger population from which the sample is taken.

Once you take measurements, you are left with many numbers or scores (called *data*). The next step is to make sense of the numbers. You do this by organizing and describing the distribution of the data. Only then can you test your hypothesis by conducting a test for statistical significance to ultimately answer the research question (reject or not reject the hypothesis).

EXAMINING RAW DATA

The first step is to look at the original, or raw data—for the purpose of this discussion—and describe them. Do not perform any mathematical operations yet. To fully describe the data, you must first clean and organize them.

CLEANING DATA

Cleaning data means making sure no scores are missing and that scores are entered into the spreadsheet and computer correctly. The set of numbers may be incomplete or incorrect; for example, a decimal point may be in the wrong place. In a sense, by cleaning the data, you can see them more clearly (metaphorically, there is less dirt on them) and therefore notice whether all data are present and accounted for. Mistakes can easily be made in a study if the investigator is careless and enters the data incorrectly into the computer or if there is a bug in the software that corrupts the data.

For example, when you examine your bank statement, you notice an error on the bank's part. Perhaps you were charged a fee by mistake or the bank did not record one of your transactions. These data-entry errors have to be identified. Researchers working with spreadsheets must never confuse blank cells that represent missing data, such as a subject's refusal to answer, with zeros that have been interpreted as low scores by the computer.

ORGANIZING DATA

When you first collect data (measure and record information from a subject), they are unsorted and likely to be unintelligible. If you cannot understand the data, you certainly will not be able to see any interesting patterns and trends in them. It is only after we "gain control over seemingly chaotic data"[1(p46–47)] and start to see patterns in the data, that progress in science is made.

For example, when it sends your monthly statement, the bank has organized your checks by date. By looking at this organized statement, you may notice trends in when you pay your bills. You may notice that you pay most of your bills at the end of the month but that you wait an extra week before paying the electric bill. Perhaps you hate the electric company and feel it probably deserves to be paid last. This pattern may have become obvious to you only once your check-writing history was presented to you in an organized way.

Organizing data usually means ranking all the collected scores for a group performance from lowest to highest and then counting how frequently each value occurs in the group. This is called a *frequency distribution* and is easily accomplished with a computer or even by hand. After the scores are organized, you can begin to appreciate how the group behaved and whether any outstanding or extreme values are present. For example, if deposits in your checking account are organized by amount from smallest to largest, you may more readily notice an extreme value at the bottom of the statement (called an *outlier*), such as a $25,000 deposit that probably was a mistake.

Another way to organize data are by sorting them into "bins" on the basis of some characteristic, such as individuals treated versus those not treated.

DISPLAYING DATA: A PICTURE IS WORTH 1000 DATA POINTS

Once organized, values can be displayed graphically for better visualization of the data. The idea is that a picture is worth 1000 words (or in this case 1000 numbers). Another way of saying this is that by graphing the data, you see the big picture.

All the scores as a group can be reduced visually to three important summary values—average score for the group (central tendency), spread of the values (variability), and the symmetry of the distribution. By viewing a data graphically, researchers can identify important patterns, errors in data collection, noise in the data (variability), and outliers. It can be argued that looking at the "pictures" can yield far more information than the much-revered test of the hypothesis.[2,3]

FREQUENCY DISTRIBUTION

You can plot a frequency distribution, which takes each score and plots a bar the length of which corresponds to the number of times that score occurred (Figure 10-1). This tells you how frequently scores occur in your sample. By tradition, for nominal data, bar graphs are used (there are spaces between the bars). For interval and ratio and frequently for ordinal (rank) scores, histograms (Figure 10-2) are used (no separation between adjacent bars).

BOX AND WHISKER PLOTS

A second popular way of displaying data are with a box-and-whisker plot (also called *box plot*). In some formats, the middle value indicates the median, the outside borders of the box indicate the middle 50% of the distribution, and the whiskers mark the highest and lowest scores in the distribution that are not considered outliers. Finally, the location of outliers often is indicated with circles (minor outliers) and asterisks (extreme outliers). If you look at a box plot sideways (see Figure 10-10 later in the chapter; turn the book on its side), the plot resembles the image of cat whiskers.

DESCRIBING DATA

We also need to describe the data numerically. The problem with describing data are that usually there are too many numbers. Trying to present all of them would be like trying to describe every color value in a Van Gogh sunflower painting. There are just too many. It may be easier simply to summarize the scope of yellows and purples chosen by the artist and to mention the predominate hue. By reducing the data to a few summary statistics, you can better understand, manage, and communicate information.[4,5]

Important things to remember when you view a distribution of scores are to observe (1) on average, where all the scores fall within the distribution, (2) how far each score deviates from this central location, and (3) the symmetry of the curve. These three characteristics of the distributions, which together describe the "personality" of data, are called the *average score (central tendency), spread (variability),* and *shape.*

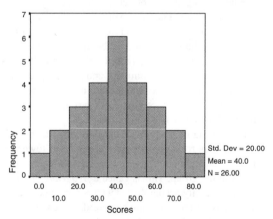

Std. Dev = 20.00
Mean = 40.0
N = 26.00

Figure 10-1.   Histogram displays how frequently a score or interval of scores occurs.

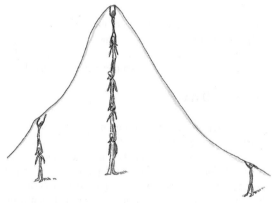

Figure 10-2.   A histogram can be envisioned as an imaginary tent formed by subjects standing on each other's shoulders to hold up the canvas. The peak or mode locates the most frequently occurring score.

CENTRAL TENDENCY: A POINT IN THE DISTRIBUTION

The central tendency is the point in the distribution where all scores tend to cluster. It is a focal point for the distribution. There are three ways to measure central tendency, each of which provides different information about the center—the mean (average), median, and mode.

Mean

The mean (average) is the most commonly used measure of central tendency in journal reports and can be viewed as the center of gravity of the distribution that takes into account the value of every score in the distribution. It is the sum of values divided by the number of values. If a score is added to one end of the distribution (added weight), the mean (center of gravity) is affected and shifts in that direction. The mean is used with interval, ratio, and frequently ordinal data but never with nominal data. It is the measure of choice among researchers if the distribution is symmetric[6] and all data are accounted for.

Median

The median is the score in the middle (location) of the distribution. That is, one half of all scores lie above this score and one half lie below it. Like the mean, the median is used with interval, ratio, and frequently ordinal data but never with nominal data. Because the location of the median is not greatly influenced by extreme scores, it is researchers' measure of choice if the distribution is asymmetric, that is, skewed or lopsided.[6]

Mode

The mode is the most frequently occurring score in the distribution. It is easy to find because it is located at the peak in the distribution. The mode is the only measure for nominal data, that is, categorical data such as religion, ethnic group, or political preference,[6] and usually is used in voting or polls.[7] The mode also can be used for ordinal, interval, and ratio data.

A distribution may have more than one mode or peak. If you are studying center of gravity and include both men and women in your study, you may observe two modes because women tend to have a lower center of gravity than men do. In such cases, you would describe the distribution as *bimodal.* It may make sense to treat the two distributions separately as coming from two different populations (men and women).

Summary of Central Tendency

The *mean* is the preferred measure of central tendency because "it is the one that varies least from sample to sample of any given population."[8(p26)] The mean varies less than the median, and the median varies less than the mode. That is one of the reasons the mean is so popular in research reports. Nevertheless, you must always ask whether an extreme score is present in your data because extreme values can have an undesirably destabilizing or distorting effect on the mean.[7]

Choice of Central Tendency

Your choice of summary statistics[8] should be based on the shape of the distribution, as follows:[9]

- Mean if the distribution is normal.
- Median if the distribution is not symmetric (perhaps because of extreme scores).
- Mode to indicate most common score.

VARIABILITY: A DISTANCE IN THE DISTRIBUTION

In addition to central tendency, it is necessary to know the variability to appreciate the performance of a group. Variability is a summary score that gives an idea of how far scores fall from the average or central common score and can be seen in the width of a curve. Variability, also called *scatter* or *dispersion,* is the distance that scores spread from average performance and gives a sense of how much "noise" there is in the performance. For example, an unskilled person may have more variability or noise in his or her performance, whereas a skilled person usually has a more consistent, less variable performance. A person with a neurologic disorder such as athetoid cerebral palsy often has greater variability in performance than a healthy person of the same age. Three types of variability measures are standard deviation, interpercentiles, and range.

Standard Deviation

The standard deviation is the most commonly used measure of variability for interval and ratio measures. It is the measure of choice when the distribution is symmetric and there are no missing data. Standard deviation is commonly used with the mean and takes into account the distance of every score from the mean.[6] It may be easier to think of standard deviation as an average or summary of individual deviations from the mean.[7,8] The mathematical formula is the square root of the average squared deviation from the mean. I hope I didn't just ruin your day. Squaring makes all the deviations from the mean positive and accentuates large deviations. Calculating the square root makes the final value more meaningful, so we're not "thinking" in squared units. All we really want to know is how far above or below the mean the scores typically lie.

Interpercentiles

Interpercentiles are ranges that contain a certain percentage of the scores. For example, the interquartile range includes the middle 50% of the scores.[7] Like the median, interpercentiles are not greatly influenced by extreme scores (outliers) and is therefore the measure of choice when the distribution is asymmetric. It is commonly used with the median.

Range

The range is the largest and smallest value of the distribution (the most extreme distances) and is useful for a quick idea of variability or if you want to know the best or worst performance in the group (e.g., who finished first and who finished last). Hence the range includes only two scores from the entire sample[8] and may be quirky if there are outliers.

Summary of Variability

Of the three measures of variability, the standard deviation of the sample provides the most comprehensive and best estimate of the variability of values (the value that varies least from values for repeated random samples). The standard deviation is better than interpercentiles, and interpercentiles are better than range for estimating values for a population.[8] Be aware, however, that an extreme score (outlier) can have an undesirably destabilizing or distorting effect on standard deviation.[9]

THE BIG PICTURE: THE IMPORTANCE OF KNOWING BOTH CENTRAL TENDENCY AND VARIABILITY

One needs to know both the central tendency and the variability of a score to get a true sense of a situation. For example, a person may report having a "normal body temperature" of 98.6°F. With additional information regarding variability however, one learns that even though the person's head is very hot (in an oven) and the feet are freezing (in an ice bucket), body temperature, on average, is indeed normal (Figure 10-3).

A second example is being told that a river is, on average, 4 feet deep. When you try to cross the river, you drown (assuming you can't swim) because although the average depth is 4 feet, the depth ranges (variability) from 1 to 14 feet,[10] a detail the Parks Department failed to share with you. Without including information on variability, important information regarding an individual's or sample's wide scope of experiences is lost.

SYMMETRY: THE SHAPE OF THE DISTRIBUTION

The third characteristic of a distribution to inspect is its overall shape. When most of the scores are in the middle of the distribution and only a few are toward the tails, the distribution resembles the outline of a bell. The shape is symmetric and the distribution is called *normal* (Figure 10-4A).

If the distribution has an extreme score (outlier) at one end of the distribution, the shape of the distribution is skewed (slanted) and becomes asymmetric. This can look like a lopsided hill, a melting bell, or a wave in the ocean (Figure 10-4B, C).

Skewed Distribution

We can use a tug-of-war metaphor to better understand how an extreme score can affect the mean and result in a skewed distribution. If an equal number of people with the same strength (scores) pull on a rope in opposite

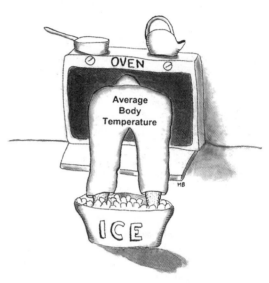

Figure 10-3. To appreciate an average value, it is helpful to know the full range of scores used in the calculation. Average body temperature, for example, can occur when all parts of a body have similar (moderate) body temperature readings or when some body parts have extreme but opposite temperatures (e.g., head in an oven, feet in a bucket of ice).

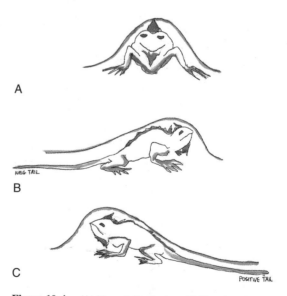

Figure 10-4. **(A)** Normal distribution. **(B)** Negative skew with left tail. **(C)** Positive skew with right tail.

directions, the middle point of the rope (average score) does not move. If a person (a giant) is added to one side of the rope, the middle point of the rope (the average score) loses the central position and moves in the direction of the extra (extreme) person (Figure 10-5).

A skewed distribution with the tail on the right side (positive skew) (Figure 10-4C) suggests that only a few individuals did very well on the test or performance. Perhaps the test was difficult. A skewed distribution with the tail on the left side (negative skew) (Figure 10-4B) suggests that only a few individuals did very poorly on the test or performance. Perhaps the test was too easy.

Measurements of reaction time are a special case. They may have markedly positively skewed distributions because of a limited scale. That is, scores can never be negative because the reaction is not measured until the subject is given a signal to which to react.

Why Is a Skewed Distribution a Bad Thing?

A skewed distribution can distort a researcher's ability to predict the behavior of a population from sample characteristics. It is therefore important to determine whether extreme scores, which can markedly contribute to a skewed distribution, are correctly collected (not a typographic error or an artifact). In the exercise at the end of the chapter, we examine the influence of extreme scores on a distribution of scores.

The Normal Distribution of Scores

The ideal distribution has a symmetric, normal, bell-shaped appearance. When randomly selected, the more subjects included in a study, the more the distribution approaches a normal curve shape. In a normal distribu-

tion, the average score lies in the middle of the curve, the variability of scores lie equally on either side of the curve, and there are no extreme scores at the tail ends of the curve. In other words, most of the scores (the most common ones) are found toward the middle of the distribution. Progressively fewer, less common scores are found as one moves farther toward either end (tail) of the distribution. When the distribution is normal, the three types of central tendencies (mean, median, and mode) agree.

In such a situation, approximately two thirds of all scores are contained within 1 standard deviation from the mean score, if the distribution of scores is bell shaped.[6,7] For example, if the mean score is 100 and the standard deviation is 15, then two thirds (66%) of all the scores within the distribution are found between the values of 85 and 115, that is, within 15 points above or below the mean. This is useful information. It means I can locate most of the scores within one unit of variation from the average score (Figure 10-6).

Furthermore, 95% (the vast majority) of scores in a normal distribution fall within two standard deviations from the mean, or in the previous example, between 70 and 130. Clinicians often use the score 2 standard deviations below the mean as a cutoff value because normally fewer than 2.5% of values are that low.

A Historical Note: What Is So Normal about the Normal Curve?

The observation that so many characteristics in life could be graphed as a bell-shaped curve of distributed scores led scientists to believe, mistakenly, that it reflected some "natural law." It was called the *normal frequency curve*.[11] In fact, the normal curve reflects chance variation.[11] As discussed in Chapter 9, if an object is repeatedly measured, all values will not be identical. Scientists agree to use the mean or average as the "true" value. Consequently, values that, for a variety of known and unknown reasons, differ from the mean value were considered *error*. Measurements that deviated slightly from the mean

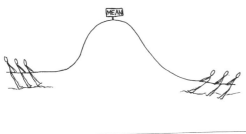

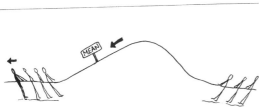

Figure 10-5. Tug-of-war. One overpowering score (*bottom, far left*) can shift the mean and cause a skew in the distribution.

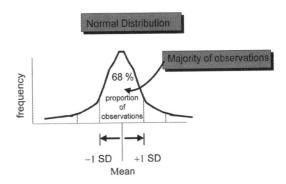

Figure 10-6. Most (68%) of the scores are found within 1 standard deviation of the average score in a normal distribution.

were viewed as small errors. Larger deviations were viewed as larger, less common errors[12] (Figure 10-7). In the early 19th century, Johann Karl Friedrich Gauss, a German mathematician, found that these errors were distributed around the mean in a symmetric, bell-shaped pattern. This distribution of "errors" in a measurement (Gauss law of errors) became known as the Gaussian distribution,[13] the normal curve of probability, or simply the normal curve.[11] In summary, the normal curve represents a distribution of unexplained or chance variation around the mean.

The Importance of the Normal, Bell-shaped Distribution

The importance of a normal, bell-shaped distribution of sample scores is that it tends to reflect the characteristics of the population from which the sample is randomly drawn. This is a good thing because you want to learn about the population characteristics but do it by studying a small sample. As a rule, at least 30 subjects in a sample are necessary to estimate population characteristics,[14] and more is usually better. Many biologic and psychological characteristics such as height, weight, and intelligence have a normal, bell-shaped appearance. Be aware, however, that some physiologic data may not be normally distributed, such as reaction times and some laboratory blood values.[13]

Some Normal Distributions in Life: The Collector

Butterflies. You like to collect things with a butterfly net. The first thing you decide to collect is, not surprisingly, butterflies. After you identify a butterfly population of interest, you proceed to randomly capture 100 butterflies, one at a time. As you observe your captured sample, you notice a pattern. Most of the butterflies

have a wingspan of 3 inches (7.5 cm), but some are smaller or larger. Fewer than 5 butterflies (5% of the sample) are either extremely large or extremely small. When you organize your sample of butterflies by size, you find that butterfly size resembles the pattern of a normal, bell-shaped distribution (Figure 10-8). As you move closer to the two tails (ends) of the bell-shaped curve, butterfly size becomes more and more extreme (tiny or huge) and less frequently observed.

Intelligence. You then say, "This is interesting. I wonder what the shape of intelligence performance would look like." Again you choose a population (persons this time) and capture 100 persons at random with, of course, a much larger net. After administering an IQ test and organizing the results, you notice a normal, bell-shaped distribution of IQ scores. To your amazement, most of the scores (average intelligence) lie within the body of the distribution. Only a few persons who have taken the test are raving geniuses or utterly unintelligent, and their scores lie on the right and left tails (ends) of the distribution, respectively.

Strength. If you test biceps strength among a randomly selected group of healthy young men, you will also probably see a pattern of scores that has a normal, bell-shaped distribution. Most young men can lift a substantial amount of weight by flexing their elbows. Fewer men can lift somewhat more or less than this load. Still fewer can lift only a small fraction (weaklings) or a large multiple of this load (muscle men).

THINGS TO DO

REVIEW DESCRIPTIVE STATISTICS USING STATISTICAL SOFTWARE

Goal

To observe how one extreme score (outlier) can affect a normal distribution of scores.

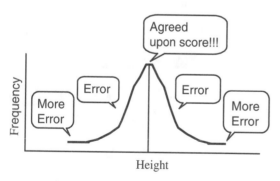

Height

Many Measurements of the Same Height

Figure 10-7. The best method of determining the "true" score of anything is to take an average of several scores. Scores on either side of this average are then viewed as error.

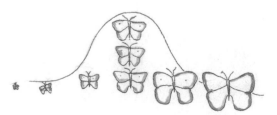

Figure 10-8. Normal distribution of butterflies. Average size is found near the center, whereas tiny and huge butterflies are located toward the tails of the distribution.

Note

The exercise is performed with Statistical Package for the Social Sciences (SPSS) for Windows version 10 (SPSS, Inc., Chicago, Ill) with step-by-step instructions, but other statistical software can easily be used. If SPSS is not available, you can use a different statistical program and the software manual or help function to guide you in conducting these analyses. Some of the statistical procedures and graphing in Chapters 10 through 12 and 23 can be conducted to a limited extent with Microsoft Excel. You need a basic knowledge of computers and Windows format. You need little or no mathematics knowledge, so relax. If none of these options is available, you may still benefit by following along.

Overview

We will do the following:

1. Enter dummy (made-up) data into a spreadsheet.
2. Examine the output of a normal distribution of scores.
3. Enter an outlier and reexamine the output to see how the extreme score affects a normal distribution of scores.

Step 1: Enter Data into a Spreadsheet

For this exercise, use the spreadsheet in SPSS. However, you can also use a spreadsheet from another software package, such as Excel, and import the data into your statistical package. The first step in examining data is entering them into a spreadsheet and checking the accuracy before analyzing the data. Menu choices are in capital letters.

1. Open SPSS.
2. Go to FILE and select NEW FILE.
3. You will see a new spreadsheet of cells (boxes) organized in rows and columns.
4. Place your cursor in the top cell of the first column (labeled VAR00001) and click on that cell.
5. Enter the following dummy data. (Press ENTER after each value; do not type the commas): 0, 40, 10, 80, 40, 10, 70, 20, 40, 70, 20, 60, 40, 20, 60, 40, 30, 50, 30, 50, 30, 50, 30, 50, 40, 60
6. There should be 26 entries in one column.
7. Go to FILE.
8. Select PRINT.
9. On the printed spreadsheet, compare the accuracy of entries with the data in number 5 above to determine whether you have made errors in entry.

Step 2: Examine the Distribution

The next step to analyzing data is to organize it. Let's say the data represent wrist extension range of motion (in degrees) among an elderly population. When you look at the data, you find it difficult to see a pattern of any kind until the data are organized from lowest to highest values.

1. Examine a histogram to determine the shape of the distribution.

a. Look at the histogram of the data to get a "picture" of a normal distribution of scores. Go to GRAPH and select HISTOGRAM. In Histogram, highlight the variable (VAR00001) on the left and move it into the box on the right using the arrow button on the screen. Click on OK.

b. Examine the output (Figure 10-9). Notice that the data in the histogram are distributed normally (a bell-shaped curve). The horizontal axis indicates scores from low (left) to high (right). The vertical axis indicates how frequently each grouping of scores occurs. In summary, the greatest frequency of scores occur in the middle of the distribution, and the frequency tapers to lower values to the left and higher values to the right.

2. Examine a box plot for the presence of any outliers.

a. Go to GRAPH.

b. Select BOX PLOT.

c. Select SIMPLE.

d. Click on the box for Data in Chart are Summaries of Separate Variables.

e. Click on DEFINE.

f. In the Define dialogue box, highlight the variable (VAR00001) (left) and move it into the box (BOX REPRESENTS) on the right of the screen. Click on OK.

g. Examine the output (Figure 10-10). The box plot can help identify outliers. The box plot consists of a box and whiskers and displays the distribution in terms of percentiles. The actual scores are to the left of the box plot. The box defines the middle 50% of the distribution. The low end of the box is the 25th percentile (score, 27.5) and the upper end is the 75th percentile (score, 52.5) of the distribution. The horizontal line within the box indicates the median (50th percentile

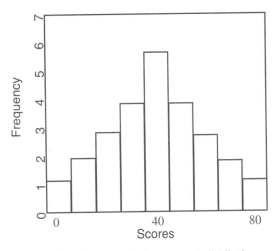

Normal Distribution of Scores

Figure 10-9. Histogram displays a normal distribution.

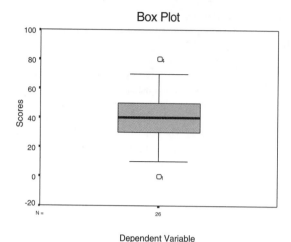

Figure 10-10. Box-and-whisker plot displays a distribution without *extreme* scores (outliers).

or middle point of the distribution) (median score, 40). The whiskers (horizontal lines above and below the box) indicate the largest and smallest values in the distribution that are not outliers. Subjects 1 and 4 (circles) are considered mild outliers because they lie above and below the whiskers.

3. Let's look at the descriptive statistics.
   a. Go to ANALYZE.
   b. Select DESCRIPTIVE STATISTICS,
   c. Select FREQUENCIES. Highlight the variable (VAR00001) on the left and move it into the box, called VARIABLE(S), on the right of the screen using the arrow button on the screen.
   d. Select the STATISTICS option button. Click on the following options: mean, median, mode, skewness, minimum, maximum, std. deviation.
   e. Click on CONTINUE.
   f. Click on OK. This starts the analysis.
   g. Examine the output of descriptive data. The output should appear on the screen after the analysis is completed. The result is as follows:

N	26
Mean	40
Median	40
Mode	40
Std. Deviation	20
Skewness	0
Std. Error of Skewness	.456
Minimum	0
Maximum	.80

The data confirm that scores are normally distributed. All measures of central tendency are the same (mean, 40; mode, 40; median, 40), and there is no significant skew. Significant skew is determined by dividing the skew value (0) by the standard error of the skew (0.456). Values less

than 2 generally are not considered a problem. In this example, the value is 0 (0/0.456 = 0) and therefore is not significantly skewed. In summary, the average amount of wrist extension, the most frequently found amount, and the amount of wrist extension in the middle of the distribution are all 40 degrees because the distribution of scores is normal.

Step 3: Enter an Outlier

Let's have some fun and examine what happens to the normal distribution when we add an outlier. We want to see whether an extreme score will change the characteristics of the normal distribution described in step 2.

1. Repeat the steps to enter data. Return to the spreadsheet and replace the value of 80 with an extreme value of 120. That is, introduce a subject with hypermobility and 120 degrees of wrist extension.
2. Repeat steps to examine the histogram (Figure 10-11). Notice how the outlier to the right of the distribution distorts the bell-shaped curve with a longer tail on the right side of the distribution. A tail to the right (in the positive direction) makes this distribution positively skewed. Also notice that although the most common score (the mode) continues to be 40 degrees, the mean may have been shifted to the right (pulled in the direction of the outlier). In other words, the center of gravity or balance point in the distribution—the mean—seems to have shifted from the center to the right.

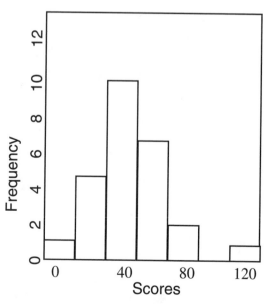

Figure 10-11. Histogram displays a positively skewed distribution caused by an extreme score (outlier). The outlier in this example has a score of 120.

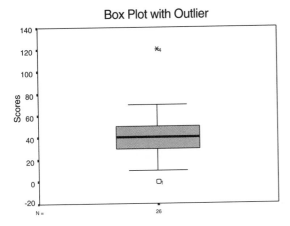

Figure 10-12. Box-and-whisker plot displays a distribution caused by an *extreme* score (outlier). The outlier in this example is a score of 120.

3. Repeat the steps for examining a box plot (Figure 10-12). Examine the box plot with the outlier. An extreme outlier is identified (subject 4 with a score of 120) in the box plot, and the extreme score does not overly affect the position of the 50th percentile (the median remains unchanged with a score of 40 degrees). In other words, the median, which is the middle point in the distribution, is not affected dramatically by an extreme score. As we will soon see, however, the mean is highly sensitive to outliers.

4. Repeat the steps for examining descriptive statistics. The result is as follows:

N	26
Mean	41.53
Median	40
Mode	40
Std. Deviation	24.28
Skewness	1.15
Std. Error of Skewness	.456
Minimum	0
Maximum	120

Although the mode and median values remain 40 degrees, the mean has changed to 41.53 degrees, pulled slightly in the positive direction toward the extreme score. The standard deviation also is larger (24.28), indicating greater variability in the data with the introduction of one outlier. The newly calculated value of the significance of the skew is 1.15/0.456 = 2.52, that is, greater than 2, and confirms that the skew is significant and therefore a problem. It is a problem because many useful statistical analyses require data that are normally distributed.

The Take-home Message

One extreme score has changed the mean value in the distribution, increased the variability, and made the distribution asymmetric. The distribution of scores no longer approximates a bell-shaped curve and became skewed.

REFERENCES

1. Sidman M. *Tactics of Scientific Research: Evaluating Experimental Data in Psychology.* New York: Basic Books; 1960.
2. Loftus G. A picture is worth a thousand p values: on the irrelevance of hypothesis testing in the microcomputer age. *Behav Res Methods Instrum Comput.* 1993; 25:250–256.
3. Wilkinson L. Task Force on Statistical Inference APA Board of Scientific Affairs. Statistical methods in psychology journals: guidelines and explanations. *Am Psychol.* 1999;54:594–604.
4. Fischer RA. *Statistical Methods for Research Workers.* 14th ed. Darien, Conn: Hafner; 1970.
5. Greenfield MLVH, Kuhn JE, Wojtys EM. A statistics primer. *Am J Sports Med.* 1996;24:393–395.
6. Moynes DR. Essential statistics review. *Am J Sports Med.* 1982;10:266–267.
7. Burrell B. *Merriam-Webster's Guide to Everyday Math: A Home and Business Reference.* Springfield, Mass: Merriam-Webster; 1998.
8. Phillips JL Jr. *How to Think about Statistics.* 4th ed. New York: WH Freeman; 1988.
9. Hartwig F, Dearing BE. *Exploratory Data Analysis.* Beverly Hills, Calif: Sage Publications; 1979.
10. Campbell SK. *Flaws and Fallacies in Statistical Thinking.* Englewood, N.J.: Prentice Hall; 1974.
11. Hillway T. *Introduction to Research.* 2nd ed. Boston: Houghton Mifflin; 1964.
12. Feinstein AR. On exorcizing the ghost of Gauss and the curse of Kelvin. *MD Comput.* 1992;9:303–323.
13. Elveback LR, Guillier CL, Keating FR Jr. Health, normality, and the ghost of Gauss. *JAMA.* 1970;211:69–75.
14. Munro BH, Page EB. *Statistical Methods for Health Care Research.* 2nd ed. Philadelphia: JB Lippincott; 1993.

11

Inferential Statistics

THE GOAL OF INFERENTIAL STATISTICS

The goal of inferential statistics is to learn about a population by estimating its characteristics from a subgroup known as a *sample*. It is called *inferential statistics* because we do not directly measure population characteristics but *infer* what we want to know about the population—our Holy Grail—from what we know about the sample. We are cheating in a sense by studying only a small sample from the population rather than studying the entire population (much more work) to learn about this population. One may want to ask, "Why study an entire herd when studying a few cows will do?"

SCIENCE, CHANCE, AND THE DEVIL

By conducting an experiment, we hope to collect reliable information (data). *Reliable* means that if the experiment were to be repeated, we would attain the same results.[1] When data are reliable (repeatable), we become more confident that they did not result haphazardly *or from chance*. Murray Sidman draws the analogy between chance and the devil: ". . . any data that cannot be proved to be independent of chance are forthwith and irrevocably assigned to its hell."[1(p43)] We try "to determine whether our data have a low probability of belonging to chance. If the data do not belong to chance, then they belong to science."[1(p43)]

DETERMINING TRUE POPULATION CHARACTERISTICS

One of the goals of researchers therefore is to ascertain, reliably, the true characteristics of a population. We usually do not know the true population characteristics but have three ways to find out.

MEASURE THE ENTIRE POPULATION

We can sample the entire population to calculate the population mean (this is rarely done and is very difficult). This would be like knocking on the door of everyone in the world who fits the criteria for the population. This clearly is not the easy solution.

CONSTRUCT A SAMPLING DISTRIBUTION

We can construct a sampling distribution to calculate the population mean. This approach is a fantasy but is crucial to understanding inferential statistics. If you were to perform the torturous task of repeatedly drawing random samples from a population, calculating the sample mean, throwing the sample back into the population, and drawing additional random samples hundreds of times, the mean (average) of all the collected sample means would equal the true population mean. The resulting distribution of all the sample means would form a normal, bell-shaped curve. The population mean (the average of all the sample means) is located in the center of this distribution. Sample means are spread out on both sides of the population mean, occurring with decreasing frequency as the tails of the curve are approached.

This normal distribution is important because researchers can estimate the true population mean by exploiting the predictive characteristics of this normal sampling distribution. For example, statisticians have found that approximately 95% of all randomly selected sample means (from our attempt to find the population mean) fall within 2 units of standard error (a measure of variability) from the true population mean.

ESTIMATE

Using inferential statistics, we can estimate the population mean (what researchers actually do). In the real world, estimation is the most practical way of learning about the population mean. Researchers estimate because they can never state with certainty the true population. One uses knowledge of the sample obtained in a study and the predictive characteristics of the normal, bell-shaped distribution of the sample means to estimate the true population mean.

Errors in Estimating the Population

Ideally we want our sample to precisely mirror the population from which we draw the sample so that we can make accurate generalizations about the population. Although we hope that the characteristics of the sample closely estimate the characteristics of the true population, not every sample mean drawn from the population is the same. Each time you draw a sample mean from the population, it can and probably does differ from the true population mean. The larger the variability of sample means from the population mean within the sampling distribution (*standard error of the mean*), the less precise is our estimation of the population mean.

Example: Heart Rates

If the average heart rate in a population is 80 beats/min, we want the sample to have an average rate of 80 beats/min. This precision rarely occurs. We are usually incorrect to some extent (e.g., the sample mean may be lower at 75 beats/min or higher at 87 beats/min). The difference between the sample mean and the population mean is called the *sampling error*. It is called *error* because the sample may not always precisely reflect the true characteristics of the population from which it was drawn. It is an error in sampling.

Researchers Have Only One Opportunity to Estimate

Researchers only have one opportunity to sample a population. They do not have the luxury or time to sample the target population hundreds of times to form a sampling distribution and take the means of all these sample means to determine the true population mean. Instead, the estimate is based on one and only one sample. There is always the possibility that this one sample will not accurately reflect the true population mean; sampling error can occur. Even when attempts are made to minimize it, sampling error can never be completely avoided.[2]

Improving Estimates of the Population

The sample mean becomes a better estimate of the population mean when we (1) increase the sample size or (2) use a sample with low variability. This relationship is clearly expressed mathematically.

$$S_{\bar{x}} = \frac{S}{\sqrt{n}}$$

When either the sample size (the denominator) increases or the standard deviation of the sample (the numerator)

decreases, the standard error of the mean (the spread of sample means around the true population) decreases. Figure 11-1 shows that when this happens, the sample means in a sampling distribution become more packed together and therefore closer to the population mean (smaller standard error). The result is that one sample mean does not differ much from another sample mean. If they do not differ greatly from one another, sample means must be closer to the true population mean. This improved estimation with a larger sample also seems intuitively true, because the more individuals included from the population, the more the sample tends to possess the characteristics of that population.

In summary, as sample size increases or variability decreases, the standard error of the mean (the standard deviation of sample means) decreases, and estimates of the true population characteristics improve. Thus we know with greater certainty (although never 100% certainty) what the population mean is within limits. It is noteworthy that populations known to have highly variable characteristics (e.g., some neurologic disorders such as Huntington's disease) may necessitate use of a larger sample size in research because a smaller sample may not adequately represent such a population.[2]

Estimating the Population Mean with a Certain Level of Confidence

When they know the characteristics of a sample (mean, standard deviation, sample size) and the predictive char-

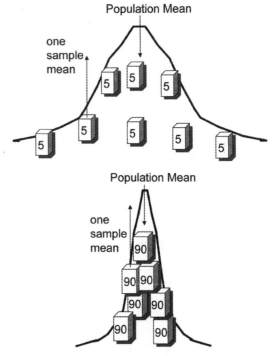

Figure 11-1. As sample size increases (e.g., from 5 to 90 subjects), sample means within the distribution come closer together and become better estimates of the true population mean.

acteristics of the normal sampling distribution, researchers can estimate with some level of confidence and within a limited range of values where the true population lies (these are called *interval estimates* or *confidence intervals* [CIs]). Researchers use CIs to estimate the characteristics of the true population.[2]

68% Confidence Interval.   We may be only a little confident that the true population mean falls within a small interval (1 standard error) of the sample mean. After all, we would need to be very precise to state that the population mean could be located within such a narrow interval of scores. We call it the 68% CI. Over the long run, one would estimate the population mean to reside within only 1 standard error of the sample mean 68 times in 100. If we were to construct 100 CIs, we would estimate from the predictive characteristics of the normal curve that 68 of these intervals would contain the true population mean.

> **Example**
> **40 (68% CI, 36.0–43.9)**

The mean score is 40, and we are 68% confident that the true population mean lies between the scores of 36 and 43.9. That is, 68% of the time the true population would be expected to fall between 36 and 43.9.

95% Confidence Interval.   We can increase our confidence a little more when we say that the true population mean falls within a wider interval (2 standard errors) of the sample mean (95% CI). Over the long run, 95 times of 100 we would estimate the population mean to lie within this larger interval of 2 standard errors from the sample mean. If we were to construct 100 CIs, we would estimate from the predictive characteristics of the normal curve that approximately 95 of these intervals would contain the true population mean. This also means that we would expect the population to lie outside this CI only 5% of the time.[2] That's rare.

> **Example**
> **40 (95% CI, 32–48)**

The mean score is 40, and we are 95% confident that the true population mean lies between the scores of 32 and 48.

99% Confidence Interval.   We may be extremely confident that the true population mean falls within an even wider interval of our sample mean (3 standard errors) (99% CI). Over the long run, we would expect the population mean to fall within this very large interval of 3 standard errors from the sample mean, 99 times in 100. That also means that we would expect the population to lie outside this CI only 1% of the time. That's extremely rare.

> **Example**
> **40 (99% CI, 29.0–50.9)**

The mean score is 40, and we are 99% confident that the true population mean lies between the scores of 29 and 50.9.

Summary: The Wider the Interval, the Lower the Precision

As the interval of the distribution in which we are willing to accept the true population mean increases, the less precise we are about the location of the true population mean. Although confidence improves with a wider interval, precision about the location of the mean is sacrificed (Figure 11-2). The following two metaphors may be helpful in understanding this concept.

Example: Bull's-eye

I am not confident that my arrow (metaphorically, the estimated population mean) will land within the innermost circle of the bull's-eye. I am much more confident that my arrow will land in a broader area anywhere on the target or on the tree from which the target is suspended.

Example: Locating the President of the United States

I am somewhat confident that I can locate the President (the estimated population mean) precisely in the West Wing of the White House (a small interval). I am more

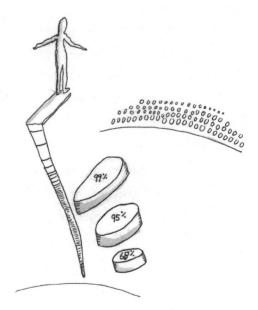

Figure 11-2.   Confidence intervals. The wider the interval, the lower is the precision. As the interval (size of the pool) of the distribution in which we are willing to accept the true population mean becomes larger (e.g., the 99% pool), the less precise we are about the location of the true population mean (e.g., where the diver actually lands in the pool).

confident that I can locate the President in the Washington, DC area (a larger interval). I am even more confident (but much less precise) that he is in the Northern Hemisphere (a huge interval).

Why Is All This Important?

This information is important because we use statistics to help determine the probability that a treatment works or does not. We are asking in statistical terms: Do the two groups in an experiment merely represent two samples drawn from the same population, or are they different enough to be considered from two different populations? That is, did the treatment make them different? To answer this question, we need to estimate the two populations means and compare them.

As a sample mean approaches the tail of the sampling distribution, the sample becomes less and less likely to be drawn randomly from the true population—the sample lies outside the 95% CI. Perhaps the mean of the sample, because of some treatment, for example, is rare enough to fall within this extreme portion of the probability curve. Although it is possible but unlikely that the sample still belongs to the original population simply because of chance (5% chance due to sampling error), a score this rare probably no longer reflects the characteristics of the original population.

Example: The Happy Pill

If you want to study the effect of a happy pill on a population, you might first draw a random sample of 30 persons because the population may be too large to study to measure their level of happiness. The resulting distribution may show most people are content (not happy and not sad), a few people are somewhat happier or somewhat less happy, and even fewer people are either euphoric or desperately depressed. In other words, the distribution is normal.

If we administer happy pills to the same sample and remeasure level of happiness, we may find that the subjects are significantly happier after the treatment than they were before the treatment. In other words, the happiness scores are so different from the original distribution of scores that the sample no longer accurately represents the population from which it was originally drawn. Such happiness would occur rarely in the original population, perhaps only 5 times in 100. We can say that in all probability, the treatment worked. That is, the sample on the posttest is statistically different from the original sample drawn from the population.

In statistical theory, as discussed earlier, it is assumed that samples are randomly selected.[2] Convenience sampling (nonrandom sampling), which is common in health care research, can limit researchers' ability to make inferences about the population from the sample because the sample may not be representative of the population.

Hypothesis Testing

Hypothesis testing is conducted to determine probabilistically whether samples are likely to belong to the same population.

Testing the Null Hypothesis. When we state a null hypothesis, we are saying that all scores come from the same population, that there are no significant differences between group scores, and that any differences (e.g., after treatment) are simply chance occurrence based on sampling error. We run a significance test to test this null hypothesis and to determine whether any differences in the samples are likely due to chance or unlikely due to chance at a given level of probability.

Analogy: The Null Hypothesis and the Justice System. The null hypothesis and justice system have similar assumptions[3,4] (Figure 11-3). In the justice system, we start with the notion that the accused is innocent. That is, he or she comes from the same innocent population as does everyone else. Because we are all fair minded, we have no reason to believe otherwise. The only way to change our minds about our belief is through the demonstration that it is highly unlikely that the person is innocent. In the courtroom, we therefore look for evidence such as fingerprints and DNA to change our minds beyond a reasonable doubt from innocence to guilt.

In the research laboratory, we start with the null hypothesis that all scores come from the same population. A score would have to fall within the improbable region (the tail region) of a normal, bell-shaped curve, where scores rarely fall, to allow us to conclude that the scores in question are probably unique.

Examining Group Differences. You can get a quick sense of differences by looking at (eyeballing) the relative distribution of scores. It can be argued that more information can be gleaned from data presented graphically than can be gleaned from a hypothesis test.[5] First look at scores for both groups at the same time. Observe whether these distributions are clearly two separate entities or whether they blend into one mass. If the groups can clearly be differentiated from each other, they may be statistically different, perhaps because of a treatment. If the two distributions seem to blend and overlap into one mass of scores, the groups may share similar scores and may not be statistically different (Figure 11-4).

Example: The Flashlight

To gain an appreciation of group differences and similarities, tape cut-outs of two bell-shaped curves (made from index cards) over the heads of two flashlights. By projecting the two lights onto the wall, you can overlap or separate the illuminated distributions. The greater the overlap of the two distributions, the more likely it is that the scores are from the same population. The less the dis-

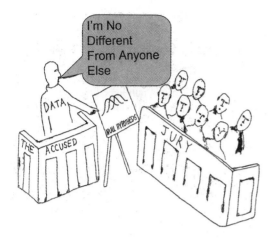

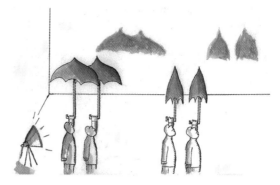

Figure 11-5. When umbrellas are folded, the silhouettes are differentiated as groups that have less variability even though the mean differences do not increase (the two umbrellas are not moved farther apart).

Figure 11-3. The null hypothesis can be thought of as the defendant in the U.S. judicial system. Researchers start by assuming the data in question are no different from any other data.

tributions overlap, the more likely it is that the scores come from different populations, perhaps demonstrating differences that are statistically significant (Figure 11-4).

Example: The Umbrella

Still another way to gain an appreciation of group differences and group variability is by having two people each fully open an umbrella and project the silhouettes of the umbrellas onto a wall. The more the two silhouettes overlap, the greater is the number of shared scores between the two groups and the less likely it is that the groups are statistically different from each other. When the umbrellas are closed, the spread decreases (less variable, less noise), making it easier to see group differences because there is less overlap between the two groups (Figure 11-5).

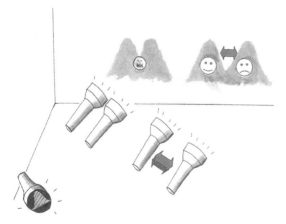

Figure 11-4. When flashlights are moved apart, mean differences increase and the illuminations become differentiated (happy and sad groups) even though the variability remains unchanged.

Testing for Significance. To objectively test a hypothesis, you need to conduct a significance test. The test is used to find the amount of variability in the scores within and within groups. If the variability between group means is comparable with the variability of scores within groups, group performances tend to overlap (they have similar scores) and do not stand out as unique from each other. Scores from all groups would tend to belong to the same population. We would say that the groups are not statistically different.

On the other hand, if the distance or variability in scores between group means is greater than that within each group, group performance may stand out as unique (less overlap of scores from the different groups). Perhaps the overlap of scores exists only at the tail ends of each distribution, where scores from each group are much less likely to occur. We would say that the groups are statistically different. A significance test confirms this difference at a given probability level. In other words, a test of significance is used to determine whether differences are so extreme that the value is unlikely to have occurred by chance.[2] A significance test provides a P value.

The P Value: What Does It Mean? The "final common pathway"[6(p202)] of all tests of significance is the P value, for probability. The P value indicates the likelihood that an observation occurs by chance alone. When we say $P = .05$, we mean the likelihood of finding the result by chance, if no relationship exists, it is 5 times in 100. A value of $P = .006$ means the likelihood of finding the result by chance is only 6 times in 1000. That is, it has a low likelihood of occurrence. A value of $P = .98$ means that the event is likely to occur 98 times in 100 (extremely likely). The lower the P value, the less likely it is that the result can be attributed to chance (Figure 11-6). Scientists seek reliable data that have a low probability of belonging to chance. Although in most hypothesis testing $P = .05$ is used as the conventional albeit arbitrary level

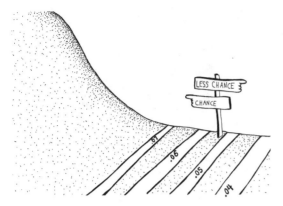

Figure 11-6. That chance is the explanation for a phenomenon is less likely as scores move closer to the tails of a distribution. In science, we are interested in events that are probably not due to chance.

for determining the cutoff between chance and statistically rare events, other probability values can be used. As Rosnow and Rosenthal put it, "surely, God loves the .06 nearly as much as the .05."[7(p1277)]

Statisticians working in industry and agriculture historically used the P value to help them make decisions. For example, the P value may have guided decisions about the use of manure in planting crops, that is, should we use manure or not?[6,8]

You Can Never Be One Hundred Percent Sure. You can never be 100% sure about your decision that two groups are statistically different (the treatment works) or that two groups remain the same (the treatment does not work).[9] This is because your decision to reject or not reject the hypothesis is based on probability (the likelihood that an event will occur), which is between 0 and 100% certainty.

You can be absolutely correct only if you test the entire population or if the probability is either 0 or 100%. Zero probability means there is no chance that something will occur; 100% probability means that occurrence is guaranteed. Most events in life are somewhere in between. Death (and taxes) and growing older are the only certain events in life—they are 100% likely to occur. It may seem to be a revelation that no matter how famous you are as an investigator or how prestigious your publication record, conclusions about your study can be wrong simply because of chance. Think about that the next time you hear an arrogant authority in the field present his or her findings at a conference.

You May Be Right. You may be right that a treatment works. This would be the same as saying, "I am going to reject the null hypothesis because I found differences. I therefore cannot support the null hypothesis that no differences exist. The intervention made the treatment group

different from the other group." Congratulations on your decision.

You may also be right that a treatment did not work. This would be the same as saying, "I am not going to reject the null hypothesis because I did not find any differences. I therefore can support the null hypothesis that no differences exist. The treatment did not make the groups different." Again, congratulations on your decision.

You May Be Wrong. Because you are making decisions based on probability, you can still be wrong in your decision even though the chances of being wrong are quite low. (Someone can say I will not win the lottery because the probability is extremely low that I will win, yet I still could win. They could be wrong.)

Two Types of Wrong Decisions

THE FALSE ALARM. The first wrong decision is that the treatment may not work and you report that it did. This is a *Type I error* or α *error*. It is a false alarm. The house is not on fire. The treatment does not work. You made the wrong decision. You said, "I'm going to reject the null hypothesis because it states there are no differences between groups, but I did find differences. I can therefore not support this hypothesis. I believe the treatment made a group different." A mnemonic device is that α is the first letter of the Greek alphabet and is the first kind of error you can commit during hypothesis testing.

The problem is that if you decide your groups are different because of the probability that groups should be expected to be different only 5 times in 100 just by chance (a low probability), it is possible that the groups are different solely because of chance (it can happen 5% of the time) and not because of treatment. You need to avoid a Type I error if the finding of the study will result in expensive interventions—the treatments may not be effective.

THE LOST OPPORTUNITY. A second wrong decision is that the treatment may be effective, and you report that it did not work. This is a *Type II error* or β *error*. You missed your finding. You win the lottery but do not collect. You made the wrong decision. You said, "I'm not going to reject the null hypothesis because it stated there would be no differences between groups, and I agree. I did not find differences. I can therefore support the null hypothesis. I believe the treatment did not make a group different." A mnemonic device is that β is the second letter of the Greek alphabet and is the second kind of error you can commit during hypothesis testing.

The problem is that you may have been able to find differences in the groups that showed the treatment was effective, but your study was not sensitive or powerful enough to pick up the differences. The power of your test was too low to detect real differences that existed. You need to avoid a Type II error if the negative findings from the study will lead to discontinuing life-saving treatment—the treatment may be effective.

Why Is β Number Two? Social Analysis of a Statistical Tradition.

Rosamond Gianutsos,[10] in a paper presented in 1975, posed the radical notion that society loses out from potentially life-saving medical discoveries, such as vaccines, because of Type II error (β error). She contended that "beta errors are number two" (α is number one) because α errors are professionally embarrassing and give scientists a "black eye" when they are wrong by stating a significant finding when none exists. Scientists thus vigilantly guard against α errors, whereas β errors, which may have greater repercussions for society, are given less attention.[10]

Trade-offs between Type I and II Errors.

There are trade-offs between Type I and II errors,[11] as there are in many aspects of research. If you reduce your risk of committing a Type II error (missed opportunity) by making your study more sensitive, your risk of committing a Type I error (false alarm) increases. The reverse also is true.[2] Like sampling error, Type I (false alarm) and Type II (missed opportunity) error can be minimized but not completely avoided.[2]

Making a Study More Powerful: Reducing the Risk of Type II Errors

The power of a study is its ability or sensitivity to detect a statistical difference when one actually exists. If you go into a dark room and are asked whether there is something in the room, you would probably report there is not because it is dark and you can't see anything. If the dimmer is turned up so that the room lights begin to shine, you are more likely to see something in the room if something is there. If the lights are turned to full brightness (the power is the highest), the likelihood of finding something in the room increases markedly. If you do see something in the room, you realize you had originally made an incorrect decision. There always had been something in the room, but you were not sensitive enough to detect its presence with the lights (power) off. As the light increases in intensity, so does the probability of finding something (Figure 11-7). By turning up the power, you increase the sensitivity of your test and therefore increase the likelihood of detecting something important, such as a significant finding, if one exists (Sharon L. Weinberg, written communication, Sept. 1999).

If you do not find statistical significance in your study, one possibility, of course, is that there simply is not any. The second possibility is that the power of your study is too low. You did not look hard enough. If a study shows no significant differences, you should always ask whether the power was too low.

Increasing the Power (Sensitivity) of a Study

The sensitivity (power) of your study can be increased in at least three ways—increasing the sample size, increasing the α level, and increasing the treatment effect.[12]

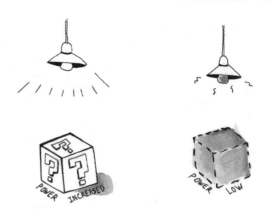

Figure 11-7. Power can be likened to a light source on a dimmer switch. The brighter you turn up the light (*left*), the more likely you will be able to detect something if it exists. The lower the power (*right*), the less likely it is that something will be detected.

Increasing Sample Size.

You can increase the number of subjects in your study (sample size). By doing so, you tend to better differentiate one group from other groups. In a high jump metaphor, one person (a small sample) may not be able to clear the bar, but several persons standing on one another's shoulders (a larger sample) may enable one of them to clear the bar and achieve statistical significance (Figure 11-8A). By increasing sample size, you reduce the standard error and improve your estimate of the true population mean. In other words, you can better detect which samples probably do and do not belong to the same population. If, however, a study has a sufficiently large sample size, any difference, no matter how trivial and unimportant, can become statistically significant.[13]

Increasing α Level.

A second way to improve sensitivity is by instituting a less stringent α level to make it easier to reject the null hypothesis. In other words, if the α level is raised from .05 (or 5%) to 10%, you are saying that any group scores that are likely to occur no more than

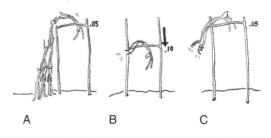

A   B   C

Figure 11-8. The high jump as a metaphor for improving the power of a study. (**A**) Increasing sample size. (**B**) Setting a less stringent α level (lowering the bar). (**C**) Increasing the effect size (adding springs to the shoes).

10% of the time by chance will be considered significant enough to say they are unique. This is a more liberal criterion than setting the α level at its more conventional 5% level. In the high-jump metaphor, a bar set too high will not be cleared. If the bar is lowered (e.g., lower the passing grade), a marginally deserving person will be able to clear the bar and reach statistical significance (Figure 11-8B).

Increasing the Treatment Effect. A third way to improve the sensitivity of a study is to use treatments (independent variables) that have a greater effect on performance measures. This is called *increasing the effect size.* If you are studying the effect of alcohol consumption on gait (walking a straight line), you may not detect the difference between a group that drinks $1/_8$ ounce (3.75 mL) of water and a group that drinks $1/_8$ ounce of vodka. However, if you increase the amount of each fluid to $1/_2$ cup (120 mL), you increase the effect size of the treatments and probably will be able to detect a sway in gait for the vodka group only. In the high-jump metaphor, testing the effects of two conventional types of sneakers may not influence high-jump performance, but using a shoe with a spring design may have a greater effect (Figure 11-8C).

Other Ways to Increase Power: Maximizing Information. Power can be increased through maximizing the amount of information or reducing the noise in the data. Ways to enhance information include (1) using a covariate to control statistically for potentially confounding variables that can cloud a relationship,[14] (2) using a repeated measures (within subjects) design to minimize the noise in the data,[11,14] (3) using measuring instruments that are precise (possess low measurement error),[14] and (4) utilizing parametric statistical analysis with interval or ratio data[14] (see Chapter 12).

Statistically Significant but Clinically Trivial

Perhaps one of the most important concepts to understand in this book is that findings from a study can be both statistically significant and clinically trivial.[9] That is, the treatment result may not have occurred by chance but may be of so little importance that the clinician may *not* want to apply the result to his or her patients. It is important to remember that the P value indicates not the strength of the relationship or the extent of a difference[6] (Figure 11-9) but only whether findings were not likely due to chance.

For example, if the flexibility of an experimental group improves statistically ($P < .05$) more than that of a comparison group but the improvement is tiny (4 degrees), is it really that important? This issue becomes more important when you realize that if you examine enough subjects, you can probably achieve statistical significance for just about anything. It is important to know not only whether statistical significance is attained but also whether it is important. That is, can it be applied in the clinic? Clinical importance usually is a judgment call.[15]

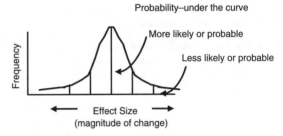

Figure 11-9. Statistical significance and effect size should not be confused. The former refers to the reliability of data (not a chance occurrence) and the latter to their magnitude.

Another example is examining the relationship between level of intelligence and shoe size among 10 adults. There should be no relationship, and the associated P value should not be statistically significant. If you reexamine the relationship but rather than 10 adults enroll 600 adults, the P value may be statistically significant even though the relationship remains unchanged, that is there is no relationship. Given enough people, a trivial relationship can turn out to be statistically significant. This feat is demonstrated in a computer exercise at the end of Chapter 12.

Report the Effect Size. One way to report the clinical importance of data is to report effect size. It is the impact of the treatment on the outcome. It indicates the extent to which the null hypothesis is false.[16] As Jacob Cohen stated, "Effect-size measures include mean differences (raw or standardized), correlations and squared correlations of all kinds, odds ratios, kappas—whatever conveys the magnitude of the phenomenon of interest appropriate to the research context."[8(p1310)] For example, if the mean difference between two originally equivalent groups is 30 pounds (13.5 kg) of force after treatment, the effect size is simply 30 pounds. This information provides more meaningful information than simply reporting that statistical significance was found (P value).

DESCRIPTIVE VERSUS INFERENTIAL STATISTICS

Sometimes researchers become so caught up in statistical significance and hypothesis testing in a study (Will the effect in the observed sample hold up when replicated?), for which they need inferential statistics, that they lose sight of the primary need to describe their data by applying descriptive statistics. Fortunately, modern computer technology allows convenient graphic tools to supplement the data description with frequency distributions and scatter plots. As shown in the exercises in Chapter 10, these tools can be sobering when you find how much a difference or relationship is affected by a single unusual data point (outlier). The message is, spend time exploring descriptive data and "looking at the pictures" graphically before diving into inferential statistics.[5,17]

THE LIMITATION OF STATISTICS

Statistics are about samples from populations and average performances,[18] not individual behavior. Clinicians will be the first to point out that knowing the results of a study does not tell them about their individual patients. Even when a patient is told an operation has a 90% success rate, that does not mean that this patient will benefit from surgical treatment. The patient may or may not benefit. It simply means that over the long run, if the operation is performed 100 times (which the patient will obviously not opt to do), the patient stands to benefit from surgery 90 times—hardly practical information from the patient's point of view.

Claude Bernard tells the humorous story of a physiologist who wanted to analyze "average European urine." He accomplished this by collecting all the urine from a railroad station urinal frequented by Europeans from many nations. The averaged physiologic, physical, and chemical characteristics of the urine collected, however, did not exist in real life.[19]

THINGS TO DO

REVIEW BASIC CONCEPTS WITH STATISTICAL SOFTWARE

Goal

To demonstrate the principles of CI. (If necessary, review the comments about software in the introduction to the exercise in Chapter 10.)

Overview

We will do the following:

1. Enter dummy data onto a spreadsheet. (Use the data from Chapter 10.)
2. Discover how using a larger CI reduces precision in estimating population characteristics.
3. Observe how increasing sample size improves the precision of estimating population characteristics.

Step 1: Enter Data onto a Spreadsheet

The first step in examining data is entering them into a spreadsheet.

1. Open SPSS.
2. Go to FILE.
3. Select NEW FILE.
4. Enter the following dummy data: 0, 40, 10, 80, 40, 10, 70, 20, 40, 70, 20, 60, 40, 20, 60, 40, 30, 50, 30, 50, 30, 50, 30, 50, 40, 60. The data represent wrist exten-

sion in degrees. (Note: If you are using the data entered in the second exercise in Chapter 10, make sure you change the score of 120 back to a score of 80 before you conduct the following analysis). There should be 26 entries.
5. Go to FILE.
6. Select PRINT. Print the spreadsheet and compare the accuracy of entries with the data from number 4 above. (Errors in data entry can occur).

Step 2: Use Error Bars (Graphs) to Compare 68%, 95%, and 99% Confidence Intervals

We want to determine how precise we can be in estimating the true population mean value of wrist extension (in degrees) from our sample.

1. Go to GRAPH.
2. Select ERROR BAR.
3. Click on SIMPLE.
4. Click on Summaries of SEPARATE VARIABLES.
5. Click on DEFINE.
6. In the DEFINE SIMPLE ERROR BAR dialog box, highlight the variable (left side of screen), and use the arrow button to move the variable (VAR00001) into the Error Bar Box on the right side of the screen.
7. Scroll through BARS REPRESENT and select CONFIDENCE INTERVAL FOR MEAN.
8. In LEVEL, type "95" in the box. (Do not type the quotation marks.)
9. Click on OK. This starts the analysis and graph construction.
10. Go to FILE, and choose PRINT to print the output of the error bar graph.
11. Repeat 8 through 10 for displaying and printing 99% CI and 68% CI. In the DEFINE SIMPLE ERROR BAR dialog box, delete "95" and type "99" in the LEVEL box and click on OK. Repeat for the 68% CI. PRINT both graphs so you have a total of three printed error bar graphs.
12. Examine the output for the three CIs (error bars) (Figures 11-10 through 11-12). The bars look like vertical whiskers with horizontal bars at each end. The two horizontal bars enclose the interval of scores (located on the left of the graph) where the population mean may lie. The three error bars have different widths. The 99% CI had the widest interval and the 68% CI has the narrowest interval.

Interpretation

99% CONFIDENCE INTERVAL.   We are extremely confident (likelihood 99 times in 100) that the true population mean will lie in a large interval of scores (i.e., scores from the 20s to the 50s). That is, we estimate that mean wrist extension of the true population is between the high 20s and the low 50s (degrees) (Figure 11-10).

95% CONFIDENCE INTERVAL.   We are highly confident (likelihood of 95 times in 100) that our true population

99% Confidence Interval

Sample size = 26

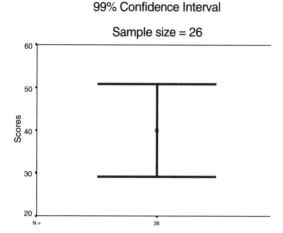

Figure 11-10. We are 99% confident (likelihood of 99 times in 100) that our population mean will lie in a large interval of scores (scores from the high 20s to the low 50s).

mean lies in a somewhat more restricted interval of scores (scores from the low 30s to the high 40s) of possible means for that population. That is, we estimate that mean wrist extension of the true population is in the range of degrees between the low 30s and the high 40s (Figure 11-11).

68% CONFIDENCE INTERVAL. We are less confident (likelihood of 68 times in 100) that our population mean will lie in an even more restricted interval of scores (scores from the mid 30s to the mid 40s) as the possible means for the population. That is, we estimate that mean wrist extension of the population is between the mid 30s and mid 40s degree range (Figure 11-12).

The Take-home Message

As an interval increases, we become more sure that the population mean lies within the interval of scores. As the interval decreases, we become less confident that the population mean lies within the interval of scores.

Step 3: To Observe How Sample Size Increases the Precision of Estimating Population Characteristics

1. Go back to the spreadsheet. Highlight all the scores in the first column of data (VAR00001). Do this by clicking the first score (in the first cell), holding down the mouse button, and dragging down the column until you get to the last score (the scores will be highlighted, or darkened).
2. Go to EDITOR and click on COPY.
3. Scroll down to the last score in the column and click on in the first empty cell below that last score.
4. Go to EDITOR and click on PASTE. This will result in 26 identical scores added below the first set of 26 scores.
5. Do this (pasting) 10 more times so that the sample grows from the initial size of 26 to a new sample size of 312 (we could do more, but for the exercise we'll stop at a sample size of 312). Take your time. Just start over if you make a mistake.
6. Plot and print the error bar of the 95% CI (as in step 2) and compare the new graph (n = 312) (Figure 11-13) with the 95% CI graph from step 1, in which the sample size was considerably smaller (n = 26) (see Figure 11-11).

By adding additional scores, that is, by increasing the size of your sample, you become more precise about the

95% Confidence Interval

Sample Size = 26

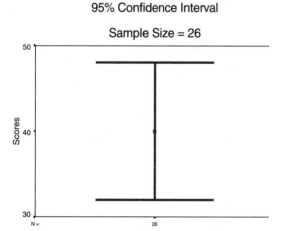

Figure 11-11. We are 95% confident (likelihood of 95 times in 100) that our population mean lies in a somewhat more restricted interval of scores (scores from the low 30s to the high 40s).

68% Confidence Interval

Sample Size = 26

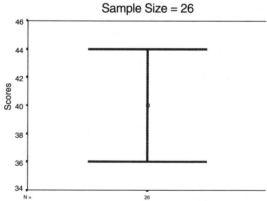

Figure 11-12. We are only 68% confident (likelihood of 68 times in 100) that our population mean will lie within a very restricted interval of scores (scores from the mid 30s to the mid 40s).

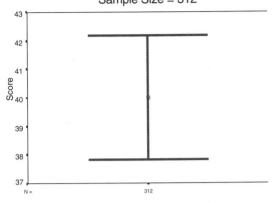

95% Confidence Interval

Sample Size = 312

Figure 11-13. We become more precise about the location of the population mean (between the scores of 38 to 42) when a larger sample size (312 rather than 26 subjects) is used.

location of the population mean. You have estimated that the population mean will lie between the scores of 32 and 48 degrees (a 16-degree interval) when the sample is fairly small (n = 26). However, when you used a larger sample size, you became more precise and located the population mean in a much smaller interval of values (between 38 and 42 degrees, a 4-degree interval). That is a 12-degree reduction in the range in which you expect the population mean to lie 95% of the time.

The Take-home Message

We become more precise about estimates of the true population mean when we add more subjects. It increases the representation of the population and reduces standard error. That is, it reduces the spread of sample means within a sampling distribution. The size of the sample in your study can affect the precision of your estimates of the true population.

REFERENCES

1. Sidman M. *Tactics of Scientific Research: Evaluating Experimental Data in Psychology.* New York: Basic Books; 1960.

2. Munro BH, Page EB. *Statistical Methods for Health Care Research.* 2nd ed. Philadelphia: JB Lippincott; 1993.

3. Kuhn JE, Greenfield MLVH, Wojtys EM. A statistics primer: hypothesis testing. *Am J Sports Med.* 1996; 24:702–703.

4. Schroeder LD, Sjoquist DL, Stephan PE. *Understanding Regression Analysis: An Introductory Guide.* Newbury Park, Calif: Sage Publications; 1986.

5. Loftus G. A picture is worth a thousand *P* values: on the irrelevance of hypothesis testing in the microcomputer age. *Behav Res Methods Instrum Comput.* 1993;25:250–256.

6. Rothman KJ. A show of confidence. *N Engl J Med.* 1978;299:1362–1363.

7. Rosnow RL, Rosenthal R. Statistical procedures and the justification of knowledge in psychological science. *Am Psychol.* 1989;44:1276–1284.

8. Cohen J. Things I have learned (so far). *Am Psychol.* 1990;45:1304–1312.

9. Baumgardner KR. A review of key research design and statistical analysis issues. *Oral Surg Oral Med Oral Pathol.* 1997;84:550–556.

10. Gianutsos R. Statistics and cognitive psychology in a social context. Paper presented at: Rutgers University; February 3, 1975; New Brunswick, N.J.

11. Portney LG, Watkins MP. *Foundations of Clinical Research: Applications to Practice.* Upper Saddle River, N.J.: Prentice Hall; 2000.

12. Cohen J. *Statistical Power Analysis for the Behavioral Sciences.* 2nd ed. Hillsdale, N.J.: L Erlbaum; 1988.

13. Cohen J. *Some Statistical Issues in Psychological Research.* In: Wolman BB, ed. *Handbook of Clinical Psychology.* New York: McGraw-Hill; 1965:95–121.

14. Light RJ, Singer JD, Willett JB. *By Design: Planning Research on Higher Education.* Cambridge, Mass: Harvard University Press; 1990.

15. Fischer EP. Art and science. *Nature.* 1997;390:330.

16. Weinberg SL, Goldberg KP. *Statistics for the Behavior Sciences.* Cambridge, Mass: Cambridge University Press; 1994.

17. Wilkinson L, Task Force on Statistical Inference, APA Board of Scientific Affairs. Statistical methods in psychology journals: guidelines and explanations. *Am Psychol.* 1999;54:594–604.

18. Hersen M, Barlow DH. *Single Case Experimental Designs: Strategies for Studying Behavior Change.* Oxford, England: Pergamon Press; 1982.

19. Bernard C. *An Introduction to the Study of Experimental Medicine.* New York: Dover; 1957.

12

Tests of Significance

Let's discuss some of the more common tests for significance used to test hypotheses in a study. Although there is a choice of inferential statistical analyses to test your hypothesis (e.g., *t* test, F test, χ^2 test), they are all tests for significance. That is, they all are used to examine whether a finding (an association or a difference) is likely to be caused by or is unlikely to be caused by chance. To quote Murray Sidman, "if the data do not belong to chance, then they belong to science."[1(p43)] The *P* value, derived from a test of significance, ultimately indicates whether data belong to chance.[2]

ANALOGY: THE INTERVIEW

It may be useful to think of the process of selecting a test of significance as a job interview (Figure 12-1). You are in a sense interviewing different statistical analyses for

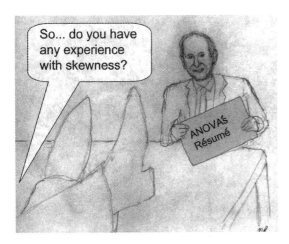

Figure 12-1. Choosing the correct test of significance is like conducting an interview. You want to "hire" the appropriate test for the job (your design and data).

the job of examining your data. As in any interview, you need to know which candidate is most suited for the job. As you would not hire an internist to operate on your hips, you also would not want to employ the wrong statistical test to analyze your data. In short, be careful about whom you hire.

The goal is to match your question and design with an appropriate statistical analysis. If a match is not attained, you can be accused of inappropriately applying a particular statistical analysis to your data, leading to results that are invalid.[3] Important considerations include the type of data (qualitative or quantitative) and the design.[3] The choice of analysis comes down to (1) applying parametric statistics to raw scores, (2) applying parametric statistics to transformed scores, or (3) using nonparametric statistics.

PARAMETRIC STATISTICS

Parametric statistics are appropriate (hire them) if quantitative (interval, ratio) and often ordinal data[4,5] are used and your data satisfy the statistical assumptions of the specific test. A common assumption is that each outcome is normally distributed (bell shaped). Be aware that if ordinal (rank) data are used in parametric analysis (a controversial issue), results should be interpreted in terms of the information in the ranked data.[3]

There are two main advantages to using parametric statistics. First, parametric statistics are powerful analyses in the sense that they exploit all the information available in continuous data.[6] That is, the data 1.6 and 2.2 contain more information than "first" or "second." This enhances the sensitivity of detecting changes in the data. The second advantage is that parametric statistics can be applied to many complex designs. It enables analyses of interaction effects, as well as the simultaneous analyses of multiple dependent variables.[7]

TRANSFORMED SCORES

If the distribution of scores is not normal (not bell shaped), the investigator must determine the reason. Often it is due to the presence of unusual scores or outliers. Errors in data entry, data from a subject admitted to the study in error (improper screening), or errors in data collection can and should be eliminated from the analysis. Data that cannot be legitimately excluded must be retained in the analysis. In either case, in the results section of the report, the researcher must reveal all decisions and actions about how data are handled. The researcher is then left to consider transforming (changing) the raw scores in the distribution to obtain a closer to normal distribution so that parametric statistical analysis can be conducted.

The reasoning behind this surprisingly acceptable practice of changing raw scores is that statistical inferences based on parametric statistics assume a normal distribution.[8] If the distribution of the sample is not normal, the statistical model may not hold true, and the analysis may be subject to error. That is, the sample statistics may not be accurate estimates of population characteristics. Because parametric analyses are considered to be robust to mild to moderate violations of parametric assumptions,[7] the concern about transforming scores is really for *gross* violations of these assumptions.

Transformations involve arithmetic operations such as squaring, finding square root, or inverting scores to make the distribution approximate a bell curve. If transformations are conducted, the type of (e.g., square root) and reason for the transformation (e.g., significant skew) should be reported in the results section of the report. Further analyses are then conducted on the transformed scores rather than the raw scores. Because transformations are decided after the fact (post hoc), replication with additional studies may support the findings.

Transformation is not recommended for every case of a lack of normal distribution, such as when the investigator can no longer interpret the meaning of the scores after the transformation.[9] For example, it may be inappropriate to transform scores derived from standardized instruments that provide normed scores for intelligence or depression because the newly transformed scales may no longer be familiar.[10]

NONPARAMETRIC STATISTICS

Nonparametric statistics do not rely on normal distribution and may be appropriate (consider hiring them) if your data are nominal (categorical) or ordinal (rank) level, the sample size is small, or the scores are not normally distributed. If a markedly skewed distribution does not respond to transformation, consider nonparametric statistics.

Nonparametric statistics have less stringent requirements about assumptions such as the distribution of your data than do parametric statistics. That is, the distribution of scores can be skewed and the sample size can be small. Although this appears to be an advantage over parametric statistics, parametric statistics are nevertheless considered robust enough to withstand moderate violations of a normal distribution of scores. *Robustness* means results will be close to accurate even if the underlying assumptions are not met.[11] (*Robustness:* I always imagine a muscle man withstanding the stormy weather on a beach even though he lacks the proper protective attire.)

Nonparametric statistics are less powerful (less likely to show significance) than parametric statistics because information is lost in the analysis. That is, continuous scores (interval) are replaced with rank scores, which provide less information.[6] This in effect reduces the sensitivity of detecting changes in the data.

In summary, parametric statistics should be seriously considered unless the data are markedly skewed (failed parametric assumptions). Consider the following list for choosing nonparametric statistics.[7]

- When no parametric alternative exists and therefore there is no parametric equivalent. For example, a χ^2 test is used to test categorical data such as disease present or disease absent.
- When data are ranked.
- When failed statistical assumptions are considered sufficiently severe, for example there are simultaneous differences in sample size and variability.
- When a short-cut calculation is needed to get a sense of the data; this need is less relevant in the computer age.

COMMON STATISTICAL TESTS: AN OVERVIEW AND INTERPRETATION

The following is an overview of the more common tests of significance, the design to which the test applies, and interpretation of the results. An extensive description of each test is beyond the scope of this book. All analyses are parametric except for the χ^2 test. Each analysis has statistical assumptions that must be satisfied before the analysis can be appropriately applied to data (see Chapter 20).

DIFFERENCES BETWEEN ACTUAL AND EXPECTED FREQUENCY (%)

χ^2 Test

The chi square (χ^2) test (pronounced *kye square,* rhymes with *high*; χ is the 22nd letter of the Greek alphabet) provides a useful nonparametric statistic obtained with a categorical level of measurement.[12] There are two χ^2 tests—goodness of fit and test for independence.

The *goodness of fit test* is used to examine whether an observed pattern of data belongs in a given distribution. You may want to know whether the frequency of hand dominance (left handed or right handed) in your sample matches, or fits, the known distribution in the population. Or you may want to know whether the frequency of blood types (O, A, B, AB) in your sample fits that in the population. If the test result is significant, the fit is said to be *poor*, meaning that the actual frequencies in your samples do not fit the expected values.

The *test for independence* (a two-way χ^2) is a test of a relationship. It is used to classify observations in two ways, such as group membership and disease, and then test whether the observations are either independent of each other or related. For example, you may want to examine whether two groups, smokers and nonsmokers, have the same likelihood of having a disease (presence or absence of lung cancer). A significant test result indicates that the categories probably are not independent and that there is a dependency in the relationship between smoking and disease. For example,

$$\chi^2 = 5.60, P = .03$$

This χ^2 value of 5.60 probably did not occur by chance because the P value is .03. Only 3 times in 100 would such a difference occur by chance.[12]

In general, χ^2 tests are used to compare actual and expected frequencies. If the difference between actual and expected frequencies is large, χ^2 is larger. A value that exceeds a critical value attains statistical significance. A significant test result would indicate a poor fit between actual and expected frequencies in a goodness of fit test or indicate a relationship between variables, such as smoking and cancer, in a test for independence.

DIFFERENCES BETWEEN TWO GROUPS

t *Test*

A *t* test is used to compare differences between two groups. An independent *t* test compares two separate groups (between-groups design), whereas a paired (dependent) *t* test is used to compare differences in the same group before and after treatment (pretest-posttest design). Statistically, we are asking whether group differences are greater than expected solely from chance. For example, you may want to compare the effect of a stressor (coffee) on an outcome (nervousness) for two groups. One group drinks coffee and the other group does not. Both groups are evaluated on a nervousness (i.e., jitteriness) scale to determine whether there is a difference in nervousness.

$$t_{1,39} = 8.45, P = .02$$

The *t* value represents the ratio of group differences (signal) to variability (noise). The numerator is the difference or separation of group (means) and therefore represents the signal or effectiveness in a treatment. The larger the numerator, the larger is the separation between the two groups (difference in nervousness) and the larger is the resultant *t* value (e.g., 8.45). The denominator in the ratio is the variability within the groups and represents the noise or spread of scores in each distribution. The more variability in the distribution in each group, the greater is the tendency for the distributions to overlap (similar scores shared by the groups). The result is less distinct separation between the groups. The larger the denominator, the greater is the within-condition variability and the smaller is the *t* value. Smaller *t* values are less likely to be statistically significant.

In general, the larger the *t* ratio, the more likely it is that statistical significance will be found (e.g., $P = .02$). The *t* value is compared with a critical value (found in tables or automatically compared with statistical software) to objectively determine whether the *t* value is large enough to achieve statistical significance. You can acquire a subjective sense of significant differences between groups simply by viewing (eyeballing) the relative distributions of the data on graphs.[13]

Be aware that in a highly variable group, such as coordination of movements in athetoid cerebral palsy, a much larger difference between group means (numerator) is needed to detect differences because there can be a great deal of overlap of scores (denominator).[14]

DIFFERENCES AMONG THREE OR MORE GROUPS

One-way Analysis of Variance

Analysis of variance (ANOVA) is used to compare differences among three or more groups or conditions. Rather than analyzing differences between two means (as done in the *t* test), ANOVA is used to examine the differences *among* group means. One-way ANOVA is used to evaluate only one condition, treatment, or factor called the *independent variable*. The test is sometimes called *univariate ANOVA* because one dependent variable or outcome is analyzed.

For example, you want to determine the effects of stressors (coffee condition) on nervousness (the outcome). You can analyze nervousness level in three separate stress groups. Group 1 drinks 2 cups of coffee, group 2 drinks 20 cups of coffee, and group 3 drinks 50 cups of coffee.

The Significance Test. In ANOVA, significance is tested through examination of the variability between the groups (the signal) and within each group (the noise). If the variability or spread of means in the numerator (called *between-group variance*) is the same as the spread of scores within each group being compared in the denominator (called *within-group variance* or *error variance*), the ratio, called the *F ratio* (developed by Fischer) is 1. An F ratio of 1 is an insignificant difference because the signal is no greater than the noise.

If the variability in the numerator (between-groups) is greater than the variability in the denominator (within-group), the F ratio is larger, and there is a greater likelihood that the F ratio will attain statistical significance.[14] In general, the larger the F ratio, the more likely it is that statistically significant differences will be found. By looking at the relative distributions of scores in groups, you can get a subjective sense of the data. Less overlap of distributions suggests a difference)[13] (Figure 12-2). Parenthetically, if you square the *t* value, you get the F ratio ($t^2 = F$).

Where Does the F Ratio Come From?   The F ratio is the ratio of average variation between groups to the aver-

age variation within groups. Again, we are looking at the ratio of signal to noise in ANOVA. The larger the signal, the more likely it is that the difference will be statistically significant.

F = Between mean square ÷ Within mean square
   = Signal/Noise

The numerator, called the *between mean square,* is derived from dividing the variation between groups (called the *sums of squares*) by a number called the *degrees of freedom.* Degrees of freedom are the number of comparisons that are free to vary.[15] The denominator, called the *within mean square* is derived in a similar way by means of dividing the within-group variation by its degrees of freedom. The F ratio is then calculated by means of dividing the between mean square in the numerator by the within mean square value of the denominator. A larger F ratio suggests greater variation between the groups, in the numerator, perhaps because of a treatment effect, since an effective treatment can increase the variation between those treated and those not treated.

Multiple Comparisons.   If you obtain a significant F ratio in one-way ANOVA, all you can say is that somewhere there is a statistical difference among the groups, but you don't know which groups. Multiple comparisons are then conducted to determine which groups in the experiment are statistically different from the others. If the F ratio is not statistically significant, multiple comparison tests are not necessary because no statistical differences will be found.

It may be helpful to think of multiple comparison tests as receiving a gift in a box (the significant ANOVA result) and opening the box only to find three or more smaller boxes. Your task is to determine which pair of means (gift boxes) is statistically significant (Figure 12-3); that is, which two are uniquely different from each other.

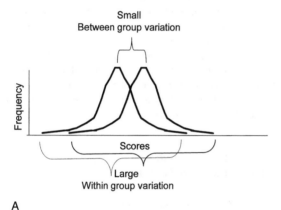

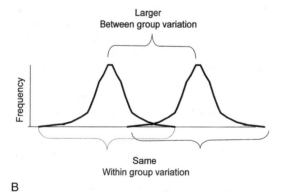

Figure 12-2.   By looking at the relative distributions of scores in groups, one can get a subjective sense of the data. (**A**) Overlapping distributions suggest no differences between groups. (**B**) Less overlap of distributions suggests greater between-group variation and possibly a statistically significant difference. Only two groups shown for illustration.

DIFFERENCES AMONG GROUPS UNDER MORE THAN ONE TREATMENT CONDITION

Two-way Analysis of Variance

Two-way ANOVA (and for that matter three-way ANOVA and higher) is used to examine group differences in more than one dimension. The advantage of two-way ANOVA is a greater approximation of real-life conditions (*enhanced external validity*) because interactions are examined (see Chapter 7).

For example, whereas the one-way ANOVA can be used to examine the effects of stressors (2, 20, and 50 cups of coffee) (condition 1) on nervousness level, a two-way ANOVA can be used to examine these same effects (condition 1) on two different groups (persons with neurosis and well-adjusted persons (condition 2). The researcher can then examine not only whether stressors

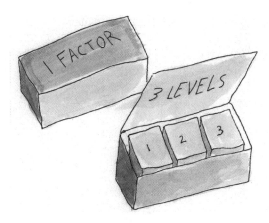

Figure 12-3. Locating where significant differences lie is like opening up a gift box only to find smaller gifts that must be opened and compared.

(condition 1) cause nervousness or whether there are group differences (between healthy persons and those with neurosis) in nervousness (condition 2) but also whether the effects of the stressor, coffee, differ depending on whether the subject is healthy or has neurosis (the interactions). This capability is important because in the clinic, you may want to know whether different types of patients will respond uniquely to the same treatment.

You test significance with two-way ANOVA by first examining differences due to interactions between the two conditions (*interaction effects*) and then looking at differences due to each condition individually (*main effects*). If statistical significance is found, you conduct multiple comparison tests to determine where statistically significant differences exist.

GROUP DIFFERENCES WITH A "NOISY" CONFOUNDING FACTOR REMOVED

Analysis of Covariance

Analysis of covariance (ANCOVA) is an extension of ANOVA but has the advantage of statistically removing a variable, called a *covariate*, that may contribute noise (error) to the outcome measure. An example is studying the effect of coffee intake on nervousness but removing the effects of test taking anxiety, which also may be related to nervousness. By identifying the related, extraneous variable (test taking) and adjusting nervousness outcomes to remove the association of the confounding factor from the analysis, you reduce the error variance (noise) and make the analysis more powerful. That is, you increase the likelihood of finding differences in your groups by removing some of the contributing "noise" in your data.

ANCOVA also has been used, albeit controversially, to equate groups (make them equal) before an experiment. An example is to equate groups on initial test scores (initial scores may be related to the outcome scores) to adjust for differences in initial performance when assessing performance after an intervention. ANCOVA has been recommended in this case only if the groups are equivalent in every way except for the variable of interest (e.g., in every way but test score).[14]

DIFFERENCES IN THE SAME SUBJECT ACROSS VARIOUS TREATMENTS

Repeated Measures ANOVA

Repeated measures ANOVA is a powerful test for examining differences in the performance of each subject across several treatment conditions (*repeated measures design, within-subject design*). In a sense, the test is an extension of the paired or dependent *t* test because it is used to compare variation (signal to noise) in the same group before and after a treatment but then takes additional measurements after additional treatments. Thus the subject's performances are repeatedly measured and analyzed. The analysis, which is used with repeated measures designs, is attractive to clinicians because it answers questions about how subjects (patients) would respond under various conditions.[14]

In an experiment that involves examining the effects of coffee intake on nervousness, rather than assigning each subject to one of three separate groups, each subject receives all three treatments but not at the same time. A subject may first drink 2 cups of coffee then undergo measurements of nervousness then after a period of time, drink 20 cups of coffee and undergo the measurements of nervousness again, and finally drink 50 cups of coffee and undergo measurements of nervousness once more. Thus the subject's outcome (nervousness) is repeatedly analyzed.

Repeated measures ANOVA is a powerful test because it removes the variability (noise) typically found among different individuals assigned to the same group. There is no group assignment in this design. By removing group variability as a source of variation from the analysis and having each subject act as his or her own control (less variation is found within the same individual), the test becomes more sensitive and usually requires fewer subjects.[14]

GROUP DIFFERENCES ON MORE THAN ONE OUTCOME

Multivariate ANOVA

Multivariate analysis of variance (MANOVA) is used to examine group differences. Rather than looking at differences in only one outcome, as is done with univariate ANOVA, the investigator looks at differences in two or more outcomes (*dependent variables*) simultaneously. For example, to examine the effects of coffee intake on both blood pressure level and nervousness, MANOVA would be an efficient way to analyze the data. The less attractive approach (univariate ANOVA) requires two separate analyses (one for nervousness and one for blood pressure). It is not desirable to conduct multiple analyses on the same data because doing so increases the likelihood of finding differences solely caused by chance (Type I error).

In MANOVA, if a statistical significant difference is found, separate univariate ANOVAs are conducted to determine whether the statistical significance can be found in either the first (nervousness) or second (blood pressure level) outcome. If an ANOVA result is significant, multiple comparison tests are conducted to determine which groups are statistically different. The gift metaphor can be useful in visualizing this concept.

ASSOCIATIONS BETWEEN TWO CHARACTERISTICS

Correlational Analysis

Correlational analysis, such as Pearson product-moment, captures in a single index the association, or relationship, between two variables. The association also can be observed in a scatter plot. This analysis, which is used in almost all fields, is an important step in establishing relationships between characteristics.[7,8] It may be helpful to think of correlation in terms of interdependence of variables.[15] For example, if nervousness and coffee intake are associated, then the more coffee I drink, the more nervous I may become or vice versa. Another way to ask this is, do changes in nervousness correspond to changes in coffee drinking? When one changes, so does the other one. There is interdependence.

Strength of the Association. You can acquire a subjective sense of correlation strength by looking at a scatter plot graph of the two variables. In general, the straighter the pattern of scores (called *linearity*), the stronger is the association between the two variables (Figure 12-4). The correlation coefficient can serve as an indicator of effect size (see Chapter 11).[16]

The strength of an association is expressed as a *correlation coefficient*. The Pearson product-moment correlation, one of the most common parametric statistics in health research,[10] is used as an example, as follows:

$$r = .80, P = .04 \text{ (two tailed)}, r^2 = .64, 1 - r^2 = .36$$

The r signifies that it is a Pearson correlation coefficient. The value .80 is the index and indicates the strength of the correlation. The index ranges from -1 to $+1$. Zero indicates no association between the variables, whereas 1 (either + or −) is a perfect relationship. The following guidelines are provided for interpreting the strength of a correlation coefficient: 0 to .25 means little or no association; .25 to .50 means a fair association; .50 to .75 is a good association; and coefficients greater than .75 are

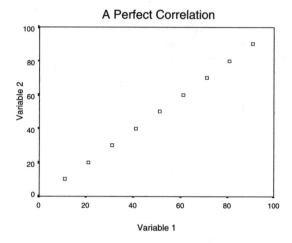

Figure 12-4. The strength of an association can be seen by looking at the pictures. A linear (straight line) pattern suggests a strong relationship, whereas a scatter of points (see Figure 12-7) suggests little or no relationship.

considered good to excellent.[17] The $r = .80$ in the equation therefore indicates a strong relationship between coffee intake and nervousness. Strength is not affected by the sign (i.e., −.80 and +.80 are equally strong).

ASSOCIATIONS AND RESTRICTED RANGE OF SCORES. The strength of an association between two variables may be deflated and not reflect the true relationship if the range of scores in the analysis is restricted, that is, if all scores are clustered together. For example, the intrarater reliability of terminal knee extension angle measurements for five knees may be low because most measurements are restricted and cluster closely around 0 degrees (e.g., 0, +2, −3, +5, 0). The strength of an association may be better reflected by including the full scope of knee angles (0, 30, 60, 90, 120 degrees).

It may be wise to anticipate the range of measures characteristic of the group you are studying before deciding a correlation analysis is appropriate. It may be more difficult to find an association in a healthy sample (whose scores may be similar and clustered together in a narrow, normal range, such as terminal knee extension) than in a clinical population (whose scores may be more varied because of pathologic conditions such as contractures). We examine the effect of restricting the range of scores during correlation analysis in a computer exercise at the end of this chapter.

Direction of the Association. The sign of the correlation indicates whether the association is positive or negative. The sign does not mean the relationship is good or bad. A positive association means that as one characteristic increases, so does the other. For example, as coffee intake increases, so does nervousness. A negative association means as one characteristic increases, the other decreases. In this case as coffee intake increases, the number of hours of sleep may decrease. (Be careful how you state the association: coffee also can have a positive relationship with number of hours awake.)

ONE-TAILED OR TWO-TAILED TEST. If a study is exploratory, that is, you are not sure that the association will be positive or negative, a two-tailed test is performed to test for statistical significance at each tail of the distribution (both the positive and the negative ends). For example, if you are not sure that coffee intake increases or decreases nervousness, you would be noncommittal, play it safe, and conduct a two-tailed test. That way, you can reject the null hypothesis if either or both associations are found to be statistically significant.

If a direction in the association is anticipated (you have a directional hypothesis based on a theory), you should consider conducting a one-tailed test. It tests only one tail of the distribution (i.e., you put all your eggs in one basket) and is considered more powerful (sensitive) than a two-tailed test. You may not want to consider a one-tailed test unless you are completely uninterested in results that run contrary to your expectations.

Significance of the Association. The P value indicates whether the relationship is statistically significant from no relationship (that is, one not simply due to chance). If the relationship is not significant (e.g., $P = .06$), the strength of the correlation coefficient does not matter because the relationship probably occurred by chance anyway: In this example, however, $P = .04$ indicates that such a relationship would only occur 4 times in 100 and therefore probably did not occur by chance.

Meaningfulness of the Association. A word is needed about the *meaningfulness* of an association (*coefficient of determination*). By squaring the r value (r^2), you indicate the percentage of one characteristic explained by variation in another characteristic. (Technically, it is the proportion of variance accounted for.) In other words, r^2 represents the percentage of variation in the dependent variable that can be explained by variation in the independent variable.[18]

If $r = .80$, then $r^2 = .64$ (64%). That is, coffee intake (the independent variable) can explain or predict 64% of the nervousness phenomenon (the dependent variable).[14] The coefficient of determination therefore is a useful and meaningful summary value because it helps to explain the variation found in life. The value r^2 can serve as a measure of effect size[16] (see Chapter 11). The complement $(1 - r^2)$, is the variation yet to be explained (36% in the example). In science, our goal is to explain everything, that is, all physical phenomena.

In a humbling "fictitious" example for aspiring PhDs, if the strength of an association between years of education and accumulated wealth is poor ($r = .25$), the proportion of variance accounted for in the association that would help predict wealth from educational level would be very small ($r^2 = .0625$, or 6%), whereas the variance left to be explained would be huge ($1 - r^2 = .9375$, or 94%).

Correspondence versus Agreement. A good correlation does not necessarily mean agreement or the attainment of identical (equivalent) scores. Even with perfect correlations ($r = 1$), scores are not necessarily identical.[15] The relationship only shows correspondence. If you want to evaluate both *correspondence and agreement* between scores, consider using an intraclass correlation coefficient (ICC).[17]

INTRACLASS CORRELATION COEFFICIENT

The ICC is a reliability coefficient and is used to examine the *agreement* (similarity) in pairs of scores in addition to their correspondence (which is done with the Pearson correlation). It is useful for evaluating the reliability of measuring instruments.[15,19]

All measurements are considered to have two components—(1) the true variation of the object (the phenomenon of interest, such as true variations between persons) and (2) the variation of the observer or instrument, which is attributed to measurement error (a bad thing). The ICC is used to examine the variation (variance) in these two components of a score; that is, ANOVA is used in the calculation.[15]

Like the Pearson correlation coefficients, ICC values range from −1 to +1. When all the variation in a score is due to measurement error, ICC = 0. When the measurement error component of the variability of a score approaches zero, the ICC becomes closer to 1 or −1, that is perfect reliability.[15] An example is as follows:

$$\text{ICC } (2,1) = .50, P = .02$$

The ICC value indicates the strength of the reliability index. The P value indicates the probability that the index value occurred by chance. In the example, an ICC of .50 indicates only fair reliability, and the P value of .02 indicates that the value is statistically significant, that is, it is probably not due to chance.

There are six formulas (1, 1; 1, k; 2, 1; 2, k; 3, 1; 3, k) for ICC depending on the goals of the analysis.[17] Model 2 (2, 1 or 2, k) is used to assess rater reliability if the goal is to generalize findings to the larger population of raters not directly assessed in the study. Model 3 (3, 1 and 3, k) is used when this goal of generalization is not important. For example, you simply want to know the reliability of your particular clinicians working your own clinic.[17] If averaged rather than individual scores are used in the calculation, then 1, k; 2, k; or 3, k models are used.

There are two main advantages to using the ICC. First, the ICC can be used to examine both agreement and correspondence. The Pearson correlation is used to examine only correspondence. Let's say you want to examine how well two clinicians estimate, without using a timer, duration of standing (in seconds) for five patients. In the following example, both the ICC (ICC [2,1] = 1.0) and the Pearson correlation coefficient (r = 1.0) indicate perfect reliability between the two clinicians' estimates; that is, the scores of the two clinicians correspond and agree.

Clinician A estimates 1 s, 2 s, 3 s, 4 s, 5 s

Clinician B estimates 1 s, 2 s, 3 s, 4 s, 5 s

The situation changes if clinician A's estimates are 3 times longer than clinician B's estimates, as follows:

Clinician A estimates 3 s, 6 s, 9 s, 12 s, 15 s

Clinician B estimates 1 s, 2 s, 3 s, 4 s, 5 s

Pearson correlation, which measures correspondence, still indicates perfect reliability (r = 1.0) because the set of times continues to show excellent interdependence (the scores correspond). The ICC, however, indicates poor reliability (ICC [2,1] = .25) because the times are no longer identical (they do not agree).

A second advantage of using the ICC is that an investigator can analyze more than two sets of scores at the same time (e.g., variables A, B, and C). For example, with the ICC, you can compare overall reliability among three or more clinicians. Pearson correlation, however, is limited to examining one pair of scores at a time (e.g., variable A and variable B, or the reliability of two clinicians). ICC is discussed because of its popularity in some specialties, such as physical therapy. It is used far less in other specialties, however. A MEDLINE search of more than 4000 abstracts published in the *New England Journal of Medicine* in a 5-year period (1995 through 1999) revealed no hits for ICC. See Chapter 23 for procedures in calculating ICC with SPSS software.

ASSOCIATION BETWEEN TWO CHARACTERISTICS WITH ANOTHER CONFOUNDING CHARACTERISTIC REMOVED

Partial Correlation

Partial correlation is used to quantify the association between two characteristics but removes the association of another characteristic from the relationship. If you are studying the effects of coffee intake on nervousness, and it is Mother's Day (the in-laws are visiting), the in-laws also may be contributing to nervousness. If you only want to analyze the association between coffee intake and nervousness, you remove the confounder, mother-in-law, from the analysis. An example is as follows:

$$r_{123} = .50, P = .0001$$

In this example, the partial correlation coefficient indicates that the relationship between characteristic 1 and characteristic 2 is moderately strong (r = .50) once the influence of characteristic 3 (in-law visit scores) is statistically removed from the analysis. The subscripts 1 and 2 are the variables of interest, and 3 is the variable removed from the analysis. The P value of .0001 indicates that the test is statistically significant. This is extremely rare; the event would occur by chance only 1 in 10,000 times.[14]

ASSOCIATION AMONG SEVERAL INDEPENDENT VARIABLES AND ONE DEPENDENT VARIABLE

Multiple Correlation

Multiple correlation is an extension of the correlation coefficient whereby additional independent variables (characteristics) are included in the analysis to help explain the association with the dependent variable (the outcome measure), for example

$$R = .90; P = .001, R^2 = .81$$

The multiple correlation is designated by a capital R, indicating that strength of the relationship of all the independent variables with the dependent variable. R values range from 0 to +1 (there are no negative R values). The R value of .90 in this example indicates an excellent relationship, although not a perfect one.

The P value of .001 indicates that the probability that this multiple correlation would occur by chance is rare (1 in 1000) and may therefore be considered statistically significant.

The R^2 value (the coefficient of multiple determination),[18] a measure of *meaningfulness*, indicates the percentage of variation in the dependent variable that can be explained by the independent variables. For example, if coffee intake, mother-in-law visits, and negative stock market reports are the three independent variables, together (when weighted) they explain 81% of the nervousness (the dependent variable).[14]

EQUATION TO MAKE PREDICTIONS FROM ONE PREDICTOR

Simple Linear Regression

Once a correlation (association) is established between two characteristics, we can develop an equation (called a *regression equation*) that enables us to predict, or estimate, the score on one characteristic if we are provided with the score on the other characteristic. Predictions are important because we try to make them in life every day (e.g., graduations, weather, earthquakes).

Correlations and Prediction

The stronger the correlation (relationship), the more accurate is the prediction. To have a perfect prediction, we need a perfect correlation ($r = 1$ or $r = -1$). For example, if there is a strong correlation ($r = .80$) between coffee and nervousness, we can develop an equation that we can use to predict (with some error, because it is not a perfect correlation) how nervous one would become if they drank a certain amount of coffee. In fact, the coefficient of determination (r^2) indicates the accuracy of the prediction. A value of $r = .80$ yields $r^2 = .64$ (64%). This means we have 64% of the information needed to make an accurate prediction in the score of the dependent variable, nervousness.[17]

Prediction versus Cause and Effect

The word *prediction* (and for that matter *correlation*) does not necessarily mean *causation*.[18] The coffee is simply associated with the nervousness. Another factor, such as the tobacco that I always smoke when I have my coffee, actually may cause my nervousness. Or perhaps the nervousness causes the smoking, which then leads to the coffee drinking. The point is, just because I can predict associations with a regression equation does not mean I have identified the source. The phenomenon is said to occur because of *interdependence*. An experiment usually is needed to demonstrate the cause.[7,9,20]

Equation of Prediction

$$y' = a + bx$$

Parts of the Equation.   The prediction (regression) equation consists of y', the predicted score; x, the predictor; b, the regression coefficient; and a, the constant. The regression coefficient (b) indicates how much the predicted score (y') changes with a change in the predictor (x).

How to Make a Prediction.   To predict a new score (y'), one simply multiplies the predictor (x) by the regression coefficient (b) and adds a constant value (a). The stronger the correlation between x and y, the more accurate is the prediction of y when x is entered into the equation.

$$y' = 3 + 0.5 \, (10)$$
$$y' = 3 + 5$$
$$y' = 8$$

In this example, if x is number of cups of coffee, and I have 10 cups, I can predict (with some error because the correlation is not perfect) a score of 8 on my nervousness scale. If I have 100 cups, the predicted nervous score is 53.

EQUATION FOR MAKING A PREDICTION FROM MULTIPLE PREDICTORS

Multiple Regression

Once we can develop a multiple correlation between a group of independent variables (multiple predictors) and the dependent variable, we can develop an equation to make predictions from the multiple predictors (called *multiple regression*). Adding useful predictors can improve the accuracy of prediction or estimation.[14] In summary, multiple regression can improve your prediction. The equation is as follows:

$$Y' = a + bx_1 + bx_2 + bx_3$$

where Y' is the predicted score; a, the constant; x, predictors, and b, weights called *regression coefficients*. For example

$$Y' = 3 + .5(10) + 1(4) + 2(10)$$
$$Y' = 3 + 5 + 4 + 20$$
$$Y' = 32$$

If x_1 is coffee (10 cups), x_2 is cigarettes (4 packs), and x_3 is mother-in-law visits (10 visits), the predicted nervousness score Y' for this person is 32.

The b weights entered into the equation are provided for each predictor (they indicate the change of Y' with a change in x) and are tested for statistical significance to ensure they contribute significantly to the prediction.

A meaningful value (β) is provided for each predictor to indicate the unique association between each predictor with the prediction; that is, they are actually partial correlations.

COMMON PARAMETRIC VERSUS NONPARAMETRIC STATISTICS

The following is a review of possible ways to analyze data with parametric or nonparametric tests. The two approaches have similar goals.[14]

To examine the relationship between two characteristics

- Parametric: Pearson product-moment coefficient
- Nonparametric: Spearman rank correlation coefficient

To compare two groups

- Parametric: t test
- Nonparametric: Mann-Whitney U

To compare two or more groups

- Parametric: ANOVA
- Nonparametric: Kruskal-Wallis H

To compare same group before/after treatment

- Parametric: Paired t test
- Nonparametric: Wilcoxon matched-pairs signed rank test

To compare same group repeated under different conditions

- Parametric: Repeated measures ANOVA
- Nonparametric: Friedman matched samples

THINGS TO DO

REVIEW BASIC CONCEPTS
USING STATISTICAL SOFTWARE

Goal

To conduct a correlation analysis. We will also examine the effect of a limited range of scores and a huge sample size on an association.

Overview

We will do the following:

1. Conduct a Pearson product-moment correlation analysis
2. Restrict the range of scores in the correlation analysis to determine its effect on the correlation
3. Observe how increasing sample size can make the correlation statistically significant although the strength of the correlation does not change.

Exercise 1: Conducting Correlation Analysis

Step 1: Enter Data into a Spreadsheet
1. Open SPSS.
2. Go to FILE.
3. Select NEW FILE.
4. Enter the following dummy data in two columns. The data represent joint angles (in degrees) of shoulder abduction, perhaps in frozen shoulders, obtained with two different measuring instruments, such as a goniometer and an inclinometer. We want to determine how well the scores obtained with the two instruments correspond. There should be 10 entries in each column.

   Column 1 (VAR00001): 35, 45, 56, 66, 72, 79, 80, 100, 124, 178
   Column 2 (VAR00001); 50, 47, 40, 75, 60, 80, 50, 110, 126, 171

5. Go to FILE.
6. Select PRINT. Print the spreadsheet and compare the accuracy of entries with the data provided. (Errors in data entry can occur.)

Step 2: Conduct a Correlation Analysis
1. Go to ANALYZE.
2. Select CORRELATE.
3. Select BIVARIATE.
4. Highlight the two variables (on the left side of the screen) and use the arrow button to move the variable (VAR00001 and VAR00002) into the variable box on the right side of the screen.
5. Click on PEARSON BOX.
6. Click on TWO-TAILED TEST.
7. Click on OK. This starts the analysis. The output should read as follows:

Pearson Correlation	.9472
Sig. (2 tailed)	000
N	10

The *r* value is .9472, which indicates excellent positive correspondence between the two measuring instruments. The significance level of 000 does not mean no significance but indicates the *P* value is less than .0005; that is, it is statistically significant. N indicates that there were 10 pairs of scores in the analysis. Now let's look at the association using a scatter plot.

1. Go to GRAPH.
2. Select SCATTER.
3. Click on SIMPLE.
4. Click on the DEFINE button.
5. Highlight the variables (VAR00001) and move it into the *Y*-axis box.
6. Highlight the second variable (VAR00002) and move it into the *X*-axis box.
7. Click on OK to construct the scatter plot (Figure 12-5).

The scatter plot (Figure 12-5) shows a nearly straight-line and suggests a strong correspondence between the variables. In this example, VAR00001 is labeled *Goniometer* and VAR00002 is labeled *Inclinometer.* Larger degrees on the horizontal (*x*) axis generally correspond to larger degrees on the vertical (*y*) axis. A large range of values are included in this analysis; scores range from 35 to 178 degrees.

Exercise 2: Determining the Effect of a Restricted Range of Scores on the Correlation

Let's see what happens to the correlation and scatter plot if we restrict the range of scores from 35 to 90 degrees rather from 35 to 178 degrees, as in Exercise 1. In other words, we will not include the full range of shoulder joint

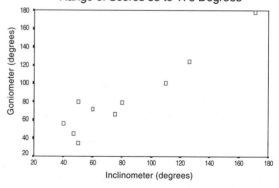

Figure 12-5. A correlation can be fully expressed when a wide range of values are included in the analysis, such as a range of shoulder mobility from 35 to 178 degrees.

values in the analysis. As you will soon see, the correlations are smaller when the range of scores is restricted.

1. Reenter the following dummy data in two columns so that the range of scores is smaller. In other words, replace the last three scores in each column as indicated:

   Column 1 (VAR00001): 35, 45, 56, 66, 72, 79, 80, 82, 87, 90
   Column 2 (VAR00001): 50, 47, 40, 75, 60, 80, 50, 83, 86, 89

   There should still be 10 entries in each column, but the scores are not as high as before.
2. Conduct a correlation analysis and construct a scatter plot again (following the steps in Exercise 1). The new output should read as follows:

Pearson Correlation	.75
Sig. (2 tailed)	.012
N	10

The *r* value is now lower at .75 and in this case indicates a strong positive correspondence between the two measuring instruments, although the strength is less now that the range of scores is more restricted (Figure 12-6).

The scatter plot (Figure 12-6) also shows a change in the distribution of scores, which are now restricted to a narrower range of joint angles. Because only a narrow range of values are included in the analysis, scores appear more clumped in the far lower left portion of the scatter plot than they do in Figure 12-5. The *r* value reflects this change (a .19 point reduction in the coefficient).

The Take-home Message. The correlation coefficient may not truly reflect the strength of the relationship of interest if the range of values used in the analysis is restricted. ICC values also are affected by a restricted range of scores in an analysis.

Exercise 3: Determining the Effect of a Huge Sample Size on the Statistical Significance of a Correlation

As discussed in Chapter 11, if you include enough subjects in your study, you can probably attain statistical significance on just about anything. This exercise may change the way you think about statistical significance; make sure you're sitting when you conduct this analysis.

Step 1: Enter the Data

1. Enter the following new data into a spreadsheet. The first set of scores represents adult IQ scores fabricated for this exercise. The second set of scores represents adult shoe size, also fabricated for this exercise. There should be 10 scores in each column.

   Column 1: (VAR00001) 10, 20, 30, 40, 50, 60, 70, 80, 90, 100
   Column 2 (VAR00002): 8, 3, 6, 9, 3, 1, 9, 5, 4, 6

2. Assuming the data were entered correctly, run a correlation analysis and a scatter plot as described in Exercise 1, step 2.
3. Observe that the scatter plot (Figure 12-7) demonstrates no relationship (no linear pattern). It is just a splatter of paired scores that looks like a Jackson Pollock painting—a canvas splattered with paint. The output should read as follows:

Pearson Correlation	–.122
Sig (2-tailed)	.738
N	10

The Pearson correlation of –.122 indicates that there is little or no relationship between intelligence and shoe

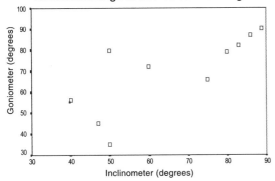

Figure 12-6. A correlation coefficient may not reflect the true relationship if the range of values in the analysis is restricted, as when a small portion of the range of motion of a joint is examined, such as shoulder mobility ranging from 35 to 90 degrees.

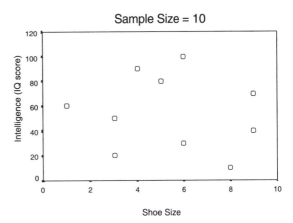

Figure 12-7. The scatter plot between intelligence and adult shoe size suggests no relationship between the variables with a sample size of 10.

size. If anything, the relationship, if there were one, would be negative. That is, the greater the IQ, the smaller would be the shoe size. The significance level $P = .738$, however, indicates that the relationship probably occurred by chance. It may occur 73 times in 100. It is not significant at $P = .05$. The analysis, however, was conducted with a very small sample, 10 subjects.

Step 2: Examine How a Larger Sample Affects Analysis. Let's see how a larger sample size affects the analysis. This is the fun part, but you need to have patience because much copying and pasting are required.

1. Go back to the spreadsheet. Highlight all the scores in the first two columns of data. Do this by clicking on the first score (first cell of the first column), holding down the mouse button, dragging to the second column, and dragging down the column until you arrive at the last score. The scores will be highlighted, or darkened. You also can hold the SHIFT key and move the arrow key rather than using the mouse.
2. Go to EDIT and click on COPY.
3. Scroll down to the last score in the first column and click in the first empty cell below the last score in that column.
4. Go to EDIT and click on PASTE. This will result in 10 identical pairs of scores added to the first set of 10 scores.
5. Repeat this process for a total of six times so that the sample grows from the initial size of 10 to a new sample size of 640. (You could do more or less, but for the exercise stop at a sample size of 640.) Take your time and don't despair because you have a large column of numbers. The copying and pasting should not take longer than 5 minutes because each block to copy and paste is twice as large as the previous one (10, 20, 40, 80, 160, 320, 640 scores). As you approach 640, keep track of how many scores you have (on the left of the screen). If you go over a little, simply highlight and delete the extra ones. As an alternative to using the mouse, you can press CTRL and the letter V (CTRL+V) as many times as needed.
6. Rerun PEARSON CORRELATION and SCATTER PLOT as described earlier.
7. Reexamine the scatter plot. It has remained unchanged from Figure 12-7 and continues to suggest no relationship even though an extremely large sample size is used (640 subjects). The new output should read as follows:

Pearson Correlation $-.122$
Sig (2-tailed)   .002
N   640

The new output confirms our suspicion that the strength of the relationship remains unchanged. An association between intelligence and shoe size remains weak ($r =$ $-.12$) even with a larger sample size (n = 640). The correlation, an indicator of effect size, remains exactly the same.

Look at the significance level. The P value is now .002. With an increase in sample size (often possible in well-funded studies), the association or lack of association becomes statistically significant.

The Take-home Message. Statistical significance, which can be achieved with large enough sample sizes, does not mean the relationship is strong or clinically important. You must always look at the meaningfulness—strength of the association (r), coefficient of determination (r^2), and magnitude of change—of data, not simply whether they are statistically significant; that is, the finding probably did not occur by chance.

REFERENCES

1. Sidman M. *Tactics of Scientific Research: Evaluating Experimental Data in Psychology.* New York: Basic Books; 1960.
2. Rothman KJ. A show of confidence. *N Engl J Med.* 1978;299:1362–1363.
3. Baumgardner KR. A review of key research design and statistical analysis issues. *Oral Surg Oral Med Oral Pathol.* 1997;84:550–556.
4. Gaito J. Measurement scales and statistics: resurgence of an old misconception. *Psychol Bull.* 1980;87:564–567.
5. Lord FM. On the statistical treatment of football numbers. *Am Psychol.* 1953;8:750–751.
6. Light RJ, Singer JD, Willett JB. *By Design: Planning Research on Higher Education.* Cambridge, Mass: Harvard University Press; 1990.
7. Cohen J. Some statistical issues in psychological research. In: Wolman BB, ed. *Handbook of Clinical Psychology.* New York: McGraw-Hill; 1965:95–121.
8. Roscoe JT. *Fundamental Research Statistics for the Behavior Sciences.* New York: Holt, Rinehart & Winston; 1969.
9. Tabachnick BG, Fidell LS. *Using Multivariate Statistics.* New York: HarperCollins College; 1996.
10. Halperin S. Spurious correlations: causes and cures. *Psychoneuroendocrinology.* 1986;11:3–13.
11. Welkowitz J, Ewen RB, Cohen J. *Introductory Statistics for the Behavioral Sciences.* 5th ed. Fort Worth, Tex: Harcourt Brace College; 1998.
12. Sternstein M. *Statistics.* Hauppauge, NY: Barron's Educational Series; 1996.
13. Loftus G. A picture is worth a thousand P values: on the irrelevance of hypothesis testing in the microcomputer age. *Behav Res Methods Instrum Comput.* 1993;25:250–256.
14. Munro BH, Page EB. *Statistical Methods for Health Care Research.* 2nd ed. Philadelphia: JB Lippincott; 1993.

15. Iverson C, Flanagin A, Fontanarosa PB, et al, eds. *American Medical Association Manual of Style*. 9th ed. Baltimore: Williams & Wilkins; 1998.

16. Cohen J. Things I have learned (so far). *Am Psychol.* 1990;45:1304–1312.

17. Portney LG, Watkins MP. *Foundations of Clinical Research: Applications to Practice*. Upper Saddle River, N.J.: Prentice Hall; 2000.

18. Schroeder LD, Sjoquist DL, Stephan PE. *Understanding Regression Analysis*. Beverly Hills, Calif: Sage Publications; 1986.

19. Shrout PE, Fleiss JL Intraclass correlation: uses in assessing rater reliability. *Psychol Bull.* 1979;86: 420–428.

20. Weinberg GH, Schumaker JA. *Statistics: An Intuitive Approach*. Belmont, Calif: Wadsworth; 1962.

13

Putting It All Together:
Matching Question–Design–Analysis

The purpose of this chapter is to help graduate students match questions, designs, and analyses in a study. The goal of the research guides these decisions. The examples are not the only way to conceive a study but are presented to foster understanding and confidence in the planning of studies.

Example

You are interested in investigating the problem of the development of pressure ulcers among users of wheelchairs.

GOAL 1

If there were absolutely nothing written on the topic, begin with a description of the problem as it affects one person or several persons.

QUESTION

What are the characteristics of a pressure ulcer? You are beginning to identify potentially important factors or variables for future studies.

DESIGN

Case report for one person, case series for more than one.

ANALYSIS

Descriptive statistics can be used for documentation. Examples are as follows:

Diameter of ulcer
Depth of ulcer
Color
Odor

Healing rates
Type of wheelchair cushion in use
Activity level of the wheelchair user
Climate (humidity)
Presence of incontinence

GOAL 2

If you have found a particular group with the problem, a description of the group is reasonable. Average characteristics of the group can be documented.

QUESTION

What are the characteristics of pressure ulcers among adults with paraplegia? You can study the characteristic identified in goal 1.

DESIGN

Descriptive (nonexperimental, observational). Cross-sectional to describe a group at one point in time. Longitudinal to describe a group over a period of time.

ANALYSIS

Descriptive statistics: means, standard deviation. You want to describe the central tendency and variability for pressure ulcers in the group.

GOAL 3

If you believe there is a relationship between some of the reported characteristics, examine the extent of the relationship.

QUESTION

Is there a relationship between activity level and healing rate? You may believe that as activity level increases to reduce ischemia from prolonged weight bearing, so will healing rate.

DESIGN

Correlational design (descriptive, cross-sectional design).

ANALYSIS

Correlational analysis (Pearson correlation) because you are seeking to associate two variables. If you believe you can predict with some accuracy healing rate from activity level because they seem to be related, consider conducting linear regression analysis. This provides you with an equation that allows you to predict healing rate from activity level.

GOAL 4

If you believe several variables are related to healing rate, include the additional variables in your analysis.

QUESTION

What is the relationship among activity level, humidity level, degree of sensory impairment, and healing rate?

DESIGN

Correlational design.

ANALYSIS

Multiple correlation, because you are seeking associations among *more than two variables*. If you can improve prediction accuracy by including these additional predictors (humidity, degree of sensory impairment), consider conducting multiple regression analysis. This provides you with an equation that allows you to predict healing rates on the basis of these three factors.

GOAL 5

If you believe diminished activity level is a *causative* factor that may lead to increased redness under the buttocks, you may start to think about designing an experiment.

QUESTION

Does weight shifting reduce erythema (redness)? That is, does a difference exist between erythema before weight shifting and erythema after weight shifting?

DESIGN

Pretest-posttest design. You measure amount of erythema, institute a weight-shifting program, and remeasure erythema status. (Without a control group or repeated measures, this is a weak design.)

ANALYSIS

Paired *t* test because you are comparing two observations for the same subjects

GOAL 6

If you believe frequency of weight shifting effects the erythema status of your patient, consider instituting three weight-shifting programs, as follows: a low-frequency program (shift weight every 2 hours), a medium-frequency program (shift weight every hour), and a high-frequency program (shift weight every 15 minutes).

QUESTION

Does frequency of weight shifting effect erythema status? That is, do differences exist in erythema status among the three weight-shifting programs?

DESIGN

Repeated measures (within-subjects design). You are repeatedly evaluating the same subjects after each intervention with sufficient time between interventions so the baseline skin condition can be reestablished.

ANALYSIS

Repeated measures analysis of variance (ANOVA) because each subject receives all interventions and you are comparing more than two observations. (A paired *t* test is used to compare two observations only.)

GOAL 7

If you believe a lack of seat cushion is a causative factor in pressure ulcer healing, you can design an experiment by introducing a cushion to an experimental group but not to an equivalent control group, both of whom have pressure ulcers. (It is generally better not to bear *any* weight over a pressure ulcer until it has healed!)

QUESTION

Does use of a seat cushion increase the healing rate of pressure ulcers more than does use of no cushion? That is, is there a difference in healing rates between the no cushion and the cushion groups?

DESIGN

Pretest-posttest control group design (also called *between-subjects design*, because you are comparing two separate groups, or *single factor design*, because you are examining only one factor [cushions]).

ANALYSIS

Independent *t* test because you are comparing two different groups.

GOAL 8

You want to evaluate three different seat cushions.

QUESTION

Do three seat cushions differ in their ability to improve the rate of healing of pressure ulcers? That is, is there a difference in healing rates for three cushion groups?

DESIGN

Multigroup pretest-posttest design (between subjects design, single factor design). There are three separate groups, one of which uses a conventional cushion.

ANALYSIS

One-way ANOVA because you are including only one factor (the cushion) and comparing more than two groups in the analysis). If you want to adjust for initial ulcer size in your comparison, consider an ANCOVA and use initial ulcer circumference as the covariate.

GOAL 9

You want to evaluate the three seat cushions but for two separate populations—persons with quadriplegia and persons with paraplegia.

QUESTION

Do the three seat cushions differ in their ability to improve rates of healing of pressure ulcers among adults with quadriplegia and those with paraplegia? That is, is there a difference in healing rate among the three cushion groups? Is there a difference in healing rate between the two populations? Does healing rate for a particular cushion depend on group membership (quadriplegia or paraplegia)?

DESIGN

Two by three factorial design, because you are comparing two population levels (paraplegia and quadriplegia) and three cushion levels.

ANALYSIS

Two-way ANOVA because you are including two factors or independent variables in the analysis—cushion and group membership (paraplegia and quadriplegia). You can examine *interaction effects* with this design.

GOAL 10

You want to evaluate three seat cushions, as in goal 8 but want to measure two different outcomes—healing rate and comfort level. That is, there are two dependent variables.

QUESTION

Do the three seat cushions differ in their ability to increase rate of healing of pressure ulcers and lead to the greatest patient comfort? That is, do differences exist in healing rates and comfort levels among the three cushion groups?

DESIGN

Multigroup pretest-posttest design (between-subjects design, single factor design).

ANALYSIS

Multivariate ANOVA (MANOVA) because you want to analyze more than one dependent (related) variable in the same study.

14

The Function of Research

Now that you've had a tour of the anatomy of a research study, it's time to learn about the function (physiology) of research—to build a more accurate view of reality.

A MORE ACCURATE VIEW OF REALITY

The ultimate function of research is to increase our knowledge so that our understanding of reality becomes richer and more accurate. This is accomplished first by acquiring new knowledge through research and then by making sense of this knowledge with theory.

CREATING KNOWLEDGE

We talk about the importance of a growing body of knowledge in the professions, but where is this "body of knowledge" anyway? For those of you who have difficulty conceptualizing a body of knowledge, go to the medical library and walk through the stacks. Knowledge is in the books, journals, dissertations, theses, and technical and government reports that fill our library shelves and continue to be updated as we continue to acquire new knowledge.

Research Creates a Mountain of Knowledge

Each experiment can be seen as *one step* in a succession of studies to better understand a phenomenon. Rarely is one experiment viewed as a seminal event that can stand on its own merits.[1] For example, Michael Faraday conducted a series of studies in a systematic manner over time to better understand electricity.[2]

The amount of knowledge on a topic accumulates as more studies are conducted in that area. If the study is free from mistakes, the results tend to be believable, and the new knowledge is added to our existing knowledge. Information gained from studies gradually develops into a mountain of knowledge. An example is the weight of evidence regarding the harmful effects of smoking; this evidence accumulated *over time*.[1]

Building a Mountain of Knowledge

Imagine that all knowledge on a subject is a mountain. As knowledge grows, the mountain becomes taller. When we climb to the top of the mountain we can see farther and gain a greater perspective on reality. If the mountain reaches to the heavens, we may even attain complete enlightenment on a subject. The goal in science is to build knowledge until all is known about a particular area.

Example: Planetary Movement and Gravity

Our knowledge of planetary motion grew gradually through the ages. The Roman Catholic Church taught that the Earth was the center of the solar system. Copernicus espoused the first well-known theory that the sun rather than the earth was the center of the solar system. His error, however, was believing that planets make circular orbits.[3,4] Kepler discovered that the planets make ellipsoid orbits around the sun rather than true circles.[4] Galileo, using a telescope, further supported the sun-centered theory of Copernicus.[4] In 1679, Newton calculated the motion of moons based on his theory of gravity, thus providing greater insight into Kepler's laws of planetary motion. We did not learn all about planetary motion in one lifetime; it took many lifetimes.

Contributing to Knowledge

New knowledge should be related to existing knowledge so that our understanding of the problem grows into a well-developed mountain rather than poorly developed, separate piles of unrelated information. Piling your knowledge on top of everyone else's knowledge produces a larger mound of knowledge. This can lead to rapid growth of knowledge in an area. Don't try to build your own, isolated pile of knowledge from the ground up (an isolated study) unless there is absolutely no information on the topic.

THEORY: MAKING SENSE OF THE MOUNTAIN

As our knowledge grows, we need to make sense of it. New theories may be proposed to provide a comprehensive understanding of reality in light of the new knowledge (see Chapter 6).

WHY DO STUDIES CONFLICT? RESEARCH, MEDIA, AND THE PUBLIC

Studies often have contradictory findings that confuse the public. Examples include conflicting reports of the benefits of oat bran in lowering cholesterol or the use of antioxidants in preventing colon cancer. The confusion may stem from exaggerated or oversimplified interpretation of research findings by the news media for the public. Clinicians understand that research is subject to mistakes, may need to be replicated, or may have limited external validity; therefore they take a conservative approach when applying results to patient care.[1]

One must view each study as work in progress that contributes a little knowledge to an overall problem. Conclusions should be viewed as tentative. They become more believable once findings are confirmed through replication.

RESEARCH AND PUBLIC POLICY

Policy decisions are influenced by the accumulation of evidence from believable (valid) studies. For example, in 1964, the connection between smoking and lung cancer led the Surgeon General to publish a government warning on smoking and to establish nonsmoking areas in public places.[5]

REFERENCES

1. Angell M, Kassirer JP. Clinical research: what should the public believe? [Editorial.] *N Engl J Med.* 1994;331(31):189–190.
2. Harre R. *Great Scientific Experiments: 20 Experiments that Changed Our View of the World.* Oxford, England: Phaidon; 1981.
3. Hart MH. *The 100: A Ranking of the Most Influential Persons in History.* Secaucus, N.J.: Citadel Press; 1987.
4. *Random House Webster's Dictionary of Scientists.* New York: Random House; 1997.
5. McGrew RE. *Encyclopedia of Medical History.* New York: McGraw-Hill; 1985.

Part III
Pathology and Vaccinations

In Part III (Chapters 15 through 20), we examine mistakes (pathologic conditions) in research that can ruin a potentially excellent study. In keeping with the boat metaphor presented in Chapter 1, these mistakes can sink your study. Part III may be particularly helpful to graduate students who are planning research.

BELIEVABILITY IN RESEARCH

The goal of researchers is to conduct a healthy, believable study. The health of a study is generally stated in terms of its validity.

VALIDITY: HOW HEALTHY IS THE STUDY?

The word *valid* means sound, convincing, well grounded, or capable of accomplishing what is intended.[1] A valid study is a sound, convincing study. The health of a study is commonly stated in terms of both *internal* and *external validity*.

Internal Validity

Internal validity means that the outcome of the study is the result of the treatment.[2] You are convinced of the results of the study under the circumstances or conditions in the laboratory. It may be useful to think of internal validity as the soundness of a study as it relates to conditions *inside* the laboratory—strictly controlled, artificial conditions (Figure III-1A).

External Validity

External validity means that the findings can be applied and are therefore sound in situations outside the laboratory, such as those in everyday life. In other words, you are convinced the results would be true under conditions you might confront in the home, in the community, with

other persons, or even at other times.[2] It may be useful to think of external validity as the soundness of a study as it relates to conditions *outside* the laboratory, in the real world (Figure III-1B). You want to know whether the finding can be applied beyond the specific context of the study, such as with other age groups and other settings (nursing homes, acute care settings).[2]

SICK STUDIES

Weak Internal and External Validity

Strong internal and external validity are desirable qualities of a healthy study. Weak studies may lack internal or external validity. In other words, mistakes by the researcher may lead one to conclude that the outcome of the study was not really the result of the treatment because confounding causes may have been introduced. The study has weak internal validity. One also can conclude that the outcome of the study cannot really be applied or generalized to the real world outside the laboratory. The study has weak external validity. Both are considered weaknesses in a study and make the results less convincing.

Strong Internal Validity with Weak External Validity

Some research is so well controlled in a laboratory that the outcome can be conclusively attributed to the treatment. The study has internal validity, but because it was conducted under the artificial conditions of a laboratory, the findings may not apply to ordinary life in the home or community. For example, the walking pattern of persons with tubes, wires, and electrodes connected to them may not reflect the gait of the same persons on a city sidewalk during rush hour (Figure III-1A, B). The study has weak external validity.

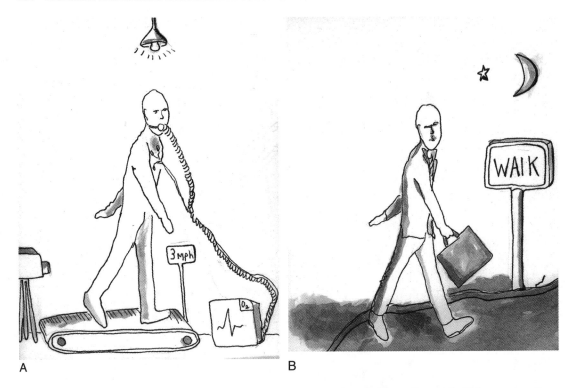

Figure III-1. (A) *Internal validity* suggests that an experiment was conducted under well-controlled laboratory conditions. (B) *External validity* suggests a study was conducted under real-life conditions.

Strong External Validity with Weak Internal Validity

Research conducted under everyday conditions (e.g., in hospital hallways, schools, community gymnasiums, or homes) may have strong external validity. Because the study lacks a controlled environment, such as protection from undesirable influences such as noise, distractions, inaccurate instruments, and nonstandardized procedures that are best controlled in a laboratory, it may be difficult to believe the results are caused solely by the intended treatment. The study lacks internal validity.

THERE IS NO PERFECT STUDY

There is no perfect study. Some studies have a great deal of internal and little external validity, and other studies have a great deal of external but little internal validity. Still other studies have weaknesses in both forms of validity.

SUMMARY

A study rarely possesses both strong internal and strong external validity. In most studies one form of validity is sacrificed to gain more of the other. One can imagine the two forms of validity as situated on opposite ends of a seesaw. In most instances, the heavier one is, the lighter the other is (Figure III-2).

An investigator needs to decide the amount of controlled as opposed to real-world environment that is to be incorporated into a research design to best answer a question. If the question can be answered in a believable way only under tight laboratory conditions, the investigator must secure internal validity at the expense of external validity. Perhaps the next study can be conducted under more real-life conditions. If the question can be answered in a believable way under realistic conditions outside the laboratory and the study can be conducted so that an unambiguous outcome can be attributed to a known cause, then securing external validity is desirable.

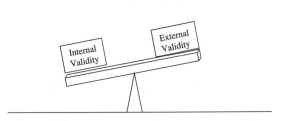

Figure III-2. Internal and external validity on opposite ends of a seesaw.

MISTAKES IN RESEARCH

Most major mistakes in research occur in the six following areas:

1. Investigator mistakes
2. Subject mistakes
3. Treatment mistakes (independent variable)
4. Measurement mistakes (dependent variable)
5. Mistakes over time
6. Mathematical mistakes (statistical mistakes).

Any of the six categories of mistakes, or biases, even if due to chance, such as sampling error and Type I or Type II error, can decrease the accuracy of results. Mistakes can lead to a less believable study. In Chapters 15 through 20, after each category of mistakes, preventive measures (vaccinations) are prescribed to help strengthen the believability (internal and external validity) of a study. See Appendix B for a complete listing of potential biases in research.

REFERENCES

1. *Webster's New International Dictionary.* 3rd ed., s.v. "validity."
2. Portney LG, Watkins MP. *Foundations of Clinical Research: Applications to Practice.* Upper Saddle River, N.J.: Prentice Hall; 2000.

15

Mistakes with the Investigator

INVESTIGATOR BIAS

Investigators are responsible for the soundness of the entire study. Because they oversee all facets of the study, investigators have a great deal of opportunity to influence findings—intentionally or unintentionally. Any preconceived notion about the outcome can influence the results. The issue of bias is even more of a concern when an investigator or a corporation funding a study has financial interest in the outcome of the study.

For example, investigators may be more enthusiastic with an experimental group and more negative with a control group (experimenter effect).[1,2] Their memory of previous subject responses, such as blood pressure reading,[2] may influence future recordings. Some investigators may be uncomfortable asking sensitive questions, such as those about sexual behavior, and this can influence how subjects respond to those questions.[2] An investigator may preferentially recruit subjects for the study (sampling bias), inject biased verbal instructions or body language that affects subject performance, or simply commit errors in math (statistical analysis) in favor of the expected outcome. In short, if you're looking for an answer, you're sure to find it. The suggestions in Table 15-1 may help protect against investigator bias and lend credibility to a study.

VACCINATION

STRICT INCLUSION AND EXCLUSION CRITERIA

The investigator should have strict criteria for admitting and excluding subjects from a study (e.g., no trauma in the past 6 months, no cognitive deficits). Initial screening of the subjects, which is typically mentioned in the methods section of a report, may be needed. By using strict criteria and screens, investigators do not have the liberty

Table 15-1. Ways to Vaccinate against Investigator Bias

- Use strict inclusion and exclusion criteria
- Employ a research assistant
- Blind the investigator
- Standardized procedures
- Provide equal attention to subjects
- Use multiple measures
- Use automated measures
- Obtain a second opinion
- Shielding the research hypothesis
- Replicate the study

to preferentially admit subjects who may help support the hypothesis, that is, prove a point.

RESEARCH ASSISTANT

Have a research assistant administer treatments and record measurements so that the investigator's biases do not influence the results. This situation may not be practical or permissible for graduate students because they need to do their own work. Under ideal circumstances, the investigator should not administer treatments (independent variable) or record the measurement (dependent variable).

While conducting experiments, assistants should be blinded from knowledge of group assignments to prevent giving extra attention to a "deprived" group. This phenomenon is called *compensatory equalization* of the groups (giving extra attention to the control group). Assistants (raters) also should be blinded to the research hypothesis so that their expectations do not influence how they take measurements.[1]

BLINDING THE INVESTIGATOR

If hiring an assistant is not possible in an experiment, the investigator should be blinded to, that is, unaware of, which subjects are in the experimental and which are in the control group. This helps to minimize unconscious cues to the subjects.[3,4]

STANDARDIZED PROCEDURES

All research personnel should follow strict, standardized procedures for administering treatments (independent variables) and recording measurements (dependent variables) to help ensure that all subjects are treated in an unbiased manner.[4] For example, instructions can be read from cue cards or tape recorded to control for potential variations in inflection or body language.

EQUAL ATTENTION

Equal amounts of time (attention) should be allocated to all groups so that attention does not become a confounding factor in your study. For example, if an experimental group receives a new treatment that is 30 minutes longer than the control condition, you may not be sure whether the treatment or the additional attention caused the improvement. Thus time becomes a confounding factor. In short, treat everyone the same way except for exposure to the experimental variable.

MULTIPLE MEASURES

If possible, multiple methods of data collection should be used in a study because results are more convincing and less likely to be influenced by bias than when only one outcome is measured. For example, if answers to a questionnaire, physical activity measurements, and range of motion recordings all support the same conclusion, none of which involves the primary investigator, findings are more convincing and less likely to have been manipulated by the investigator.

AUTOMATED MEASURES

Automated methods of collecting data should be used when possible (e.g., videotaping, audio recording, computerized data collection) rather than more subjective methods (e.g., visual observation, subjective subject report, timing with a stop watch) so that the potential for unconscious bias during data collection is minimized. For example, to time motor skills, use of a video camera that operates at 30 frames per second would be preferable to using a stop watch, which is less precise and under the operator's control.

SECOND OPINIONS

Investigators should not work alone. Other researchers should independently agree or disagree with the interpretation (meaning) of the data. For example, a study is strengthened when three impartial researchers who do not know the researcher's hypotheses or group assignments concur that gait has improved only in the experimental group. This is particularly important in measures such as gait quality or affect (mood), which are subject to interpretation.[3]

SHIELDING THE RESEARCH HYPOTHESIS

Investigators should not include their research hypotheses (expectations) in the informed consent document signed by subjects because doing so may bias the subject. This happens frequently on consent forms. Biased statements such as, "It is hoped that this treatment will reduce pain more than conventional treatments" may sink the study at the outset because subjects may either want to prove the investigator right or wrong.

REPLICATION OF THE STUDY

Repeating a study by an independent investigator (called *replication*) who reports similar results will do much to improve the credibility of the first investigator's study. Replication also can enhance the ability to generalize the findings (external validity) if a different sample or setting is used in the second study.[5] In other words, the findings from the first study are less likely due to bias or chance if similar results are reliably obtained in the second study under additional real-life conditions. Replication is the cornerstone of science.

REFERENCES

1. Portney LG, Watkins MP. *Foundations of Clinical Research: Applications to Practice*. Upper Saddle River, N.J.: Prentice Hall; 2000.
2. Gehlbach SH. *Interpreting the Medical Literature*. 3rd ed. New York: McGraw-Hill; 1993.
3. Baumgardner KR. A review of key research design and statistical analysis issues. *Oral Surg Oral Med Oral Pathol*. 1997;84:550–556.
4. Greenfield MLVH, Kuhn JE, Wojtys EM. A statistics primer. *Am J Sports Med*. 1996;24:393–395.
5. Ross LM, Hall BA, Heater SL. Why are occupational therapists not doing more replication research? *Am J Occup Ther*. 1998;52:234–235.

16

Mistakes with the Treatment

Mistakes in choosing and administering a treatment (independent variable) can threaten the credibility of a study. First, treatments must be clearly defined. If treatments are not clearly defined (operationally defined), no one will know what the investigator is actually evaluating (Is this a new piece of equipment? Do we have it in our clinic already?). Because they do not understand the treatment, other investigators will be not able to replicate the study.

Second, treatments must be administered in a consistent manner. If treatments are not administered in a consistent manner, each subject can receive a somewhat different or uncontrolled level of the independent variable. This would be analogous to giving everyone a different dosage of medication and would make it difficult to know which dosage actually caused the effect. Timing also is important in establishing causality. If treatments are not introduced at the proper times, it may be difficult to establish clearly that treatment in fact preceded the change in behavior.

Third, confounders must be identified and controlled in an experiment. Many factors other than treatment can cause a subject to improve (called *confounders*). Without control for the confounders, internal validity is compromised because there is no way to ascertain which factor caused the change.

Finally, choice of treatment can affect the external validity of a study. Experiments conducted under sterile, highly controlled laboratory conditions may not be similar to the real-life environment of the subject's home or community. For example, treatments administered by a highly trained professional may not be the same when administered by an untrained person such as a parent. Furthermore, exposing subjects to a single treatment may not simulate real-life experiences. Most patients undergo several interventions (physical therapy, occupational therapy, acupuncture), take several drugs, or have several interactions with caregivers.

VACCINATION

The suggestions in Table 16-1 may help minimize mistakes in choosing and administering a treatment (independent variable) that can threaten the credibility of a study.

COMPARISON GROUP

Internal validity is markedly enhanced when a comparison group (also called *control group*) that does not receive the experimental treatment is included in a design.[1] Comparison groups provide a baseline on which to judge the effect of a treatment on the experimental group. Without a comparison group, other factors, such as healing, remission of the disease, learning, practice, or belief that the treatment works, may unintentionally cause improvement among the subjects.

A comparison group can be given nothing, a conventional treatment, or a placebo.[2] A placebo is a treatment that is ineffective but indistinguishable to the subject and sometimes the investigator. That placebos can have a powerful effect on outcome (in medicine, one third of a wide range of treatment effects are attributed to placebos)[2] argues strongly for the need for a comparison group.

Table 16-1. Vaccination against Mistakes with Treatment

- Include a comparison group
- Standardize the treatment
- Define the treatment
- Ensure proper credentials
- Examine multiple treatments
- Increase the number of treatment levels
- Use realistic treatment settings
- Have adequate group representation
- Consider timing of treatments
- Combat the Hawthorne effect

The decision about which nontreatment to give the comparison group depends on what is being evaluated. If you want to determine whether a new treatment works, you offer the comparison group either no treatment or a placebo. If you want to determine whether a new treatment works better than a conventional treatment (often done for ethical reasons), you offer a conventional treatment to the comparison group.

STANDARDIZATION OF TREATMENTS

All persons who administer treatments (independent variables) should be trained to ensure a standardized experience.[3,4] A checklist may be useful to make sure steps in the treatment procedure are not skipped and are not delivered consistently.

Some treatments may not lend themselves to standardization. Manual therapists, for example, frequently individualize the amount or sequence of the treatment according to the unique needs of each patient. Such an approach does not ensure a similar experience for each subject and may be difficult to study experimentally. Although the method has external validity (what therapists do in the real world), it lacks internal validity (too many confounding factors may affect subject behavior because of inconsistent administration of the independent variable).

CLEARLY DEFINED TREATMENTS

Independent variables must be clearly defined in measurable, reproducible terms so that anyone can understand the intervention being evaluated (e.g., the John Doe approach, 30 minutes, 3 times a week, mornings, indoors, and in a group session). A treatment protocol in the appendix of a report can be extremely helpful to readers.

Treatments should do what they purport to do. For example, although tai chi may be used as treatment for balance, it probably would not be construed as an intensive physical activity. Misclassifying the approach can lead to inappropriate conclusions (e.g., that tai chi is useful as an intensive form of exercise).

PROPER CREDENTIALS

To improve validity, the person administering a treatment should have the appropriate credentials, such as a license or certification to practice physical therapy, medicine, or massage therapy.

EXAMINATION OF MULTIPLE TREATMENT INTERVENTIONS OR ATTRIBUTES

External validity is enhanced with a design in which investigators examine multiple treatments or different attributes (e.g., youth and advanced age) and the interactions of these treatments or attributes. Multifactorial

designs enable evaluation of interaction effects that approximate everyday life (see Chapter 7).

INCREASED NUMBER OF TREATMENT LEVELS

It is possible to increase the power (sensitivity) of a study by increasing the number of levels of treatment (independent variable).[4] Increasing the number of treatment levels gives investigators the opportunity to capture an important effect of one level.[4] For example, a study of the effect of skin pressure on motor performance that includes only low-pressure conditions may miss an important effect of a high-pressure condition.

REALISTIC, NATURALISTIC TREATMENT SETTINGS

To enhance the external validity of design, the treatment environment should be as close as possible to real life. For example, in a study of the effect of pool therapy on fitness among senior citizens living in the community, it may be more sensible to conduct the pool experience within the community, which has social benefits beyond those found in a hospital pool. Another example is having subjects participate in a tai chi class offered early in the morning at a community park, where tai chi often is practiced, rather than in a sterile, isolated, busy clinic setting.

ADEQUATE GROUP REPRESENTATION

If the independent variable is group membership (e.g., diplegia or quadriplegia; men or women), there should be sufficient numbers of subjects in each group to ensure adequate representation of each group. If some groups are underrepresented (e.g., a small number of men in the nursing profession), a stratified sampling technique can be used that takes into account disproportionate representation of subgroups within the population[4] (see Chapter 8).

TIMING OF TREATMENTS

In experiments, it is necessary to indicate clearly when treatments are delivered and withdrawn so that any ambiguity regarding the cause of an outcome can be easily resolved.[1] Withdrawal designs allow one to see whether outcomes change in one direction with treatment and change in the opposite direction when the treatment is withdrawn.

COMBATING THE HAWTHORNE EFFECT

If the Hawthorne effect—improved performance based on knowledge of being in a study—has influenced performance, determine whether the effects persist over time after the treatment is no longer administered.[4] Because it is unethical to experiment without subject consent, the Hawthorne effect is difficult to combat.

REFERENCES

1. Portney LG, Watkins MP. *Foundations of Clinical Research: Applications to Practice.* Upper Saddle River, N.J.: Prentice Hall; 2000.
2. Beecher HK. The powerful placebo. *JAMA.* 1955;159: 1602–1606.
3. Greenfield MLVH, Kuhn JE, Wojtys EM. A statistics primer. *Am J Sports Med.* 1996;24:393–395.
4. Light RJ, Singer JD, Willett JB. *By Design: Planning Research on Higher Education.* Cambridge, Mass: Harvard University Press; 1990.

17

Mistakes with the Subjects

Mistakes in managing subjects can cause a number of threats to the validity of a study. These include poor representation of the population (sampling error), unequal (nonequivalent) group assignment, small sample size, extreme groups, and personal biases of the sample[1] (Table 17-1).

POOR REPRESENTATION OF THE POPULATION (SAMPLING ERROR)

We study samples (groups of people) rather than an entire population because the population is too large a group to study. You hope the group you choose reflects the larger population of persons you ultimately want to know something about. If the sample is not randomly selected from the population, that is, if each person does not have an equal chance of being selected, you run the risk of studying a group you never intended to study in the first place (systematic sampling error). Your sample characteristics may not represent those of the true population.

Inclusion and exclusion criteria can shape the characteristics of your sample and affect the internal and external validity of your study. For example, admitting a heterogeneous sample from the population can enhance the external validity of a study because it may include the full spectrum of individuals who represent the population.[2] Use of more selective inclusion and exclusion criteria results in a more homogeneous sample and enhances internal validity.[3]

Example

Imagine you want to study the typical Manhattan dweller (the population). Rather than randomly selecting subjects, you stand on the corner of 27th Street and 1st Avenue in front of Bellevue Psychiatric Hospital to recruit them. It would not be surprising if a large percentage of the people you recruit in your study were psychiatric patients who receive treatment at Bellevue rather than typical New Yorkers.

Table 17-1. Mistakes with the Subject

Vaccination against Poor Representation of the Population

- Use random sampling
- Use a heterogeneous sample to enhance external validity
- Use a homogeneous sample to enhance internal validity
- Limit ability to generalize
- Replicate the study

Vaccination against Unequal (Nonequivalent) Group Assignment

- Randomization
- Stratify the sample
- Conduct analysis of covariance
- Avoid intact comparison groups
- Assess the damage caused by nonequivalent group assignments

Vaccination against Small Sample Size

- Conduct power analysis
- Consider the clinical importance in the power analysis
- Improve the power of the study

Vaccination against Use of Extreme Groups (Regression toward the Mean)

- Use reliable measures
- Use a comparison group
- Establish stable baseline performance
- Acknowledge limitations (possibility of regression)

Vaccination against Subject Bias

- Randomization
- Blind the subjects
- Offer desirable treatment later
- Use within-subject designs
- Ensure confidentiality

VACCINATION

Random Sampling

Random sampling enables investigators to generalize their findings beyond the sample and to the population that the sample represents[4] (see Chapter 8). The larger the sample size, the more likely it is that the sample represents the characteristics of the population.[5]

Heterogeneous Sample

To improve the external validity of the study, investigators either replicate the study with another sample that has different characteristics or use a more heterogeneous sample.[2] Selecting a target population from a wide range of settings that clinicians find relevant (hospital, nursing home, or private practice) enhances the ability to generalize the results of the study.[4]

Homogeneous Sample

To improve the internal validity of a study, investigators use a homogeneous sample with clearly delineated characteristics.[2] This typically is accomplished through stating exclusion criteria that help to narrow the population characteristics and control for extraneous factors that can confound the study.[4] For example, results of studies involving patients in a rehabilitation setting and those in a nursing home may be different because goals, environment, and social support system are dissimilar for the two groups.

Limitation of Ability to Generalize

Researchers who cannot use a design that incorporates random sampling acknowledge lack of probability sampling as a limitation of the study and apply the findings only to the sample described and to persons with the same characteristics.[5] It would be inappropriate to generalize the findings to the larger population because there is no guarantee that the sample truly reflects the population.

Replication

Studies must be replicated to determine whether findings are reliable and therefore less likely the result of sampling error.

UNEQUAL ASSIGNMENT TO GROUPS

In experiments, investigators hope to have equivalent groups when they begin the study. They want the groups to be, on average, similar in all ways except for the treatment experience.[4] This usually is attained through *randomization* whereby researchers assign subjects randomly to groups. This occurs after the subjects have been selected from the population. If the groups are not equivalent, that is, different in an important characteristic at the beginning of the study, they may respond differently,

not because of the treatment but because of the other characteristics.

VACCINATION

Randomization

The sample should be randomly assigned to groups to enhance equivalence before an experiment.[6] This works well when the sample is large. Random assignment is useful because it minimizes bias in group assignment in that assignment is due to chance rather than due to the investigator's or subjects' decisions.[4] When possible, randomization should be performed at the lowest level.[4] That is, individuals rather than intact groups (e.g., ambulation classes) and intact groups rather than intact organizations or institutions (e.g., hospitals) should be randomly assigned.

Stratification of Sample

If the sample size is small, investigators first stratify the sample according to important subject characteristics that may affect the outcome before randomly assigning the subjects to groups. This procedure may help equate groups when the sample size is small.

Analysis of Covariance

Researchers sometimes need to make statistical corrections for initial differences in group scores if randomization is not possible. This procedure is controversial (see Chapter 12).

Avoidance of Intact Comparison Groups

If possible, intact groups not participating in the study should not be used for comparison, such as a similar group studied 5 years ago. Although a persons not participating in the study may have similar characteristics to subjects in the experimental group, important differences not controlled through randomization may confound the findings. Current patients simply not interested in seeking a particular treatment may respond also differently from those who do seek the treatment.[4]

Assessment of Damage

At a minimum, investigators need to determine whether efforts to establish equivalent groups were sufficient to allow interpretation of the findings. That is, they need to determine whether selection bias was a confounding factor.[4]

SMALL SAMPLE SIZE

When a study has too few participants, there is a risk of not finding significant results—not because there aren't any, but because the power (sensitivity) of the study is too low (Type II error; see Chapter 11). Decreasing the sample size can cause greater chance fluctuations (noise) in the data so that the performance of one group cannot be differentiated from that of another, even though there may be a difference. The smaller the sample size, the less likely is precise estimation of the characteristics of the population. The question becomes, how much variability and what degree of error (imprecision) can be tolerated in the results?[7]

VACCINATION

Power Analysis

The best way to reduce the possibility of overlooking a finding (Type II error) is to conduct a power analysis to determine the number of subjects needed to detect a clinically important result if one exists. This is determined by considering the effect of a treatment (effect size), the desired sensitivity level, and the α level of the significance test. Tables in books on power analysis[8] contain this information. It also can be calculated with software designed for this purpose.

Clinical Importance and Sample Size

Clinical as well as statistical significance has to be considered in choosing a sample size. If an inordinate number of subjects is needed to detect a minuscule treatment effect, the study probably is not worth conducting. For example, if you need to evaluate 300 subjects to achieve statistical significance ($P = .05$), but the effect size (the change due to treatment) is only 1 degree of improvement in range of motion, how important is the finding? The answer is, not very important. This is probably the best advice in this book.[4]

SELECTING EXTREME GROUPS WITH EXTREME SCORES

Extreme groups (e.g., highly skilled or extremely unskilled subjects) tend to have unusually high or low scores that are unlikely to reoccur.[9] In comparisons of two groups with extreme scores, there is a tendency for each group to perform with less extreme scores on the second measurement, regardless of treatment effect. This is called *regression toward the mean* (regression effect), whereby the scores tend to fall back to the mean.[1] In comparing samples that have extreme scores, an investigator may incorrectly conclude that a lower-scoring person who scores better on a subsequent test is improving when in reality he or she may be scoring closer to the mean (a less extreme score). This is a difficult notion to understand but perhaps one that most researchers experience at some time.

Example: Good Day–Bad Day in Sports

Imagine you're a novice bowler and you go to a bowling alley one night and hit five strikes (all pins fall on all five attempts). You're obviously having a great day. Your good luck will not last long because eventually you will start playing your typical game, that is, regress downward toward your average game. Now imagine you're a nationally ranked bowler and you throw the ball into the gutter five times in a row. You're obviously having a horrible day. Your bad luck will not last long because eventually you will start playing your typical game, that is, regress upward toward your average game.

Whenever you compare two groups who perform extremely differently (e.g., high grades versus low grades, high skill versus low skill), you need to be concerned with regression toward the mean.

Clinical Example

A common clinical example of regression toward the mean is recording a high blood pressure for a person with hypertension only to find that the reading is normal on subsequent measurements.[9]

HISTORICAL NOTE: GOING BACK TO AN AVERAGE HEIGHT

The notions of regression toward the mean and regression were introduced in 1885, when Sir Francis Galton, an English scientist and cousin of Charles Darwin, became interested in heredity and related the height of offspring to that of their parents. Galton observed that the offspring of taller parents tended to be shorter than their parents and that offspring of short parents tended to be taller than their parents. The height of the offspring regressed to an average value for the population.[10,11]

There are additional disadvantages to including extreme groups in a study. First, including only extreme groups excludes the less extreme scores. This in effect reduces the full range of scores within the distribution and reduces the power of the study. Second, using extreme groups may reduce the external validity of the findings because the scores may include outliers that are not typical of a population.[4]

VACCINATION

Reliable Measuring Instruments

The more the measurements reflect the true score rather than measurement error (noise), the easier it will be to identify changes due to treatment rather than changes due to variability (changes) within the subjects.[2] The scores of subjects in extreme groups tend to regress and thus change.

Comparison Group

If it is necessary to look at treatment effects on a group with extreme scores, you may want to compare these scores with those for a control group that has similar extreme baseline scores. This shows the extent to which the improvement is due to treatment rather than regression of scores toward an average level.[12]

Stable Baseline Performance

Repeating measurements may help to establish the stability of subjects' baseline performances before introducing the treatment (independent variable). This way, researchers can see whether the first extreme performances are a "fluke" that will regress to an average performance or whether they are truly typical of the subject. If they measured a subject only once, researchers would never know whether they misjudged this first score as being truly extreme.[1]

Regression toward the Mean as a Possible Confounder

If it is necessary to use one group with extreme scores, and the group improves during the study, regression toward the mean may be a possible explanation for improvement and can be included in the discussion section of a report.

SUBJECT BIASES

Subjects who are biased, that is, have their own expectations, may respond to treatment in other than expected ways. Subjects' performance may improve if they know they are in the untreated group and want to "prove" the investigator wrong.[2] For example, suppose a researcher wants to determine whether one novel type of exercise is better than nothing at all. If the experimental group is given an exercise session and the control group is given nothing at all, members of the control group may spend extra time in the gym to compensate for the lack of treatment. Some subjects may try to respond in socially desirable ways so that they are viewed as "politically correct." Other subjects may feel resentful and intentionally perform badly.[2,4]

If subjects do not respond to questions on a survey or if they leave the study (see later), nonresponse bias may be an issue. It is not known whether the responses of those still in the study would be different from those who left the study.[4]

VACCINATION

Randomization

If there is bias in the sample, random assignment may help to distribute the bias evenly through groups.

Blinded Subjects

Subjects should be blinded to their group assignment (experimental or comparison group) and to the investigator's research hypothesis so they are less subject to biasing information.

Offer of Desirable Treatment

If appropriate, the experimental treatment can be offered to subjects in the control group when the study is terminated so that subjects are not deprived of or feel they are deprived of a potentially effective treatment.

Within-subjects Designs (Repeated Measures, Crossover)

A within-subjects design can be used if appropriate so that all subjects receive all treatments. If there are two conditions, the subjects usually undergo one treatment and then cross over in the middle of the study to receive the other treatment.

Confidentiality

Subject should be reassured that responses will not be linked with them personally so that they are free to respond honestly rather in ways they think they ought to. Confidentiality is required, and the consent form should make that clear.

REFERENCES

1. Gehlbach SH. *Interpreting the Medical Literature.* 3rd ed. New York: McGraw-Hill; 1993.
2. Portney LG, Watkins MP. *Foundations of Clinical Research: Applications to Practice.* Upper Saddle River, N.J.: Prentice Hall; 2000.
3. Nachmias CF, Nachmias D. *Research Methods in the Social Sciences.* 5th ed. New York: St. Martin's Press; 1996.
4. Light RJ, Singer JD, Willett JB. *By Design: Planning Research on Higher Education.* Cambridge, Mass: Harvard University Press; 1990.
5. Munro BH, Page EB. *Statistical Methods for Health Care Research.* 2nd ed. Philadelphia: JB Lippincott; 1993.
6. Greenfield MLVH, Kuhn JE, Wojtys EM. A statistics primer. *Am J Sports Med.* 1996;24:393–395.
7. Beveridge WIB. *The Art of Scientific Investigation.* 3rd ed. New York: Vintage Books; 1957.
8. Cohen J. *Statistical Power Analysis for the Behavioral Sciences.* 2nd ed. Hillsdale, N.J.: L Erlbaum; 1988.
9. Iverson C, Flanagin A, Fontanarosa. *American Medical Association Manual of Style.* 9th ed. Baltimore: Williams & Wilkins; 1998.
10. Welkowitz J, Ewen RB, Cohen J. *Introductory Statistics for the Behavioral Sciences.* 4th ed. Fort Worth, Tex: Harcourt Brace Jovanovich College; 1991.
11. Guilford JP, Fruchter B. *Fundamental Statistics in Psychology and Education.* 5th ed. New York: McGraw-Hill; 1973.
12. Campbell DT, Stanley JC. *Experimental and Quasi-experimental Designs for Research.* Boston: Houghton Mifflin; 1963.

18

Mistakes in Measurement

Any score is a combination of its true value and measurement error.[1,2] The true value is what we would ideally like to measure all the time. In life, however, this is never possible because there are always sources of measurement error. The best we can hope for is to reduce these sources of error in our study.

SOURCES OF MEASUREMENT ERROR

The three main sources of measurement error are (Table 18-1):

1. Inconsistency of the raters, such as poor eyesight, tremor, or changing judgments.
2. Inconsistency or inaccuracy of measuring instruments.
3. Inconsistency of the subject, such as being reactive to the measures, having changes in mood, or having a bad night's sleep.

IMPROVING THE CONSISTENCY OF THE RATER

VACCINATIONS

Training of Raters

To improve their own consistency (intrarater reliability) or their consistency with other investigators (interrater reliability),[3] researchers should undergo training before data collection. Training enables all raters to adhere to the rules when taking measurements. Training can be terminated when rates have achieved an acceptable criterion level of interrater reliability. An alternative is to determine why the raters do not agree and to correct the problem. Perhaps the problem can be traced to subtle motor impairments (tremors) or observations (visual impairment) among some of the raters.

Table 18-1. Mistakes in Measuring Instruments

Vaccination against Poor Consistency of Rater

- Train raters
- Standardize rating procedures
- Establish objective criteria for ratings
- Take averages
- Use same rater
- Use batteries of tests

Vaccination against Inconsistency and Inaccuracy in Measurement Instruments

- Establish validity and reliability of the instrument
- Check instrument before and after study
- Avoid ceiling and floor effects
- Choose sufficiently sensitive instruments
- Increase the items on the instrument
- Read the manual
- Calibrate the measuring instrument
- Use triangulation
- Check the accuracy of the software algorithms and formulas

Vaccination against Inconsistencies in the Subjects: Reactivity to Instruments and Testing

- Use posttest only control group design
- Include practice sessions
- Use passive measures

Standardized Rating Procedures

A checklist may be useful to ensure raters do not omit important steps while measuring. For example, an investigator filming head position during gait who forgets to place an identifying reflective marker on the head misses the head position data. Standardized test instructions should be given to all subjects.[3] Use of a script or instructions on a tape recorder may help to control for possible variations in the investigator's choice of words or inflection while describing the test. (Some subjects may be alienated by what they perceive as a lack of personal attention when a tape player is used.) *It is critical that subjects clearly understand the test instructions.*

Establishment of Objective Criteria

Objective criteria are needed for rating performance. What kind of performance is considered normal and what is abnormal? If several raters are evaluating quality of gait, what constitutes mild involvement and what constitutes moderate involvement? Perhaps involvement is based on the total number of parts that deviate from a standard, or maybe on the extent of the body part deviation. Whatever the criteria, all raters need to know them.

Taking an Average

Taking an average increases the reliability of measurement.[3] If more than one rater must be used in a study and these raters do not agree on the measurement despite training, it may be wise to have all raters assess every score. This approach is clinically consistent with the philosophy of obtaining a second or even several opinions to establish a reliable diagnosis.

Using the Same Rater

If interrater reliability remains poor, an alternative is to consider modifying the design so that only one person with good intrarater reliability takes all measurements. This approach is attractive clinically because it is consistent with a philosophy of continuity of care whereby the same clinician treats and observes a patient throughout a treatment program.[3]

Use of Batteries of Tests

Batteries of tests have greater reliability than individual tests just as results of a number of tests grouped together can lead to a more reliable diagnosis than can separate, individual assessment techniques.[3]

INCONSISTENCY AND INACCURACIES IN MEASURING INSTRUMENTS

VACCINATIONS

Establishment of Validity and Reliability of Measurements

Investigators need to determine the criteria validity (accuracy) and reliability (consistency) of measurements. They need to be confident that measurements are reliable so that identical phenomena can be dependably recorded. Measures should accurately reflect the true value of the thing being measured. If the instrument does not have

acceptable accuracy and reliability, it should not be used (see Chapter 9). Valid instruments must be revalidated if they are modified.

Reliability coefficients greater than .90 generally are desirable in clinical research.[2] Because reliability often depends on the specific procedures of a study and who is operating the equipment, researchers cannot rely solely on data provided by a manufacturer unless it is appropriate to the study. It is not enough to say, "The manufacturer said it was reliable." In an oral defense, a comment such as this can be fatal.

Checking the Instrument before and after the Experiment

It is good practice to check the accuracy and consistency of measuring devices both before and after a study. It is possible that the instrument became worn, loose, bent, or broken at some point during the study.

Avoiding Ceiling and Floor Effects

The instrument should have an appropriate measurement range. Measurement parameters should be matched to the type of subjects anticipated in the study so that ceiling and floor effects are avoided. For example, testing the hand grip strength of professional arm wrestlers with a strain gauge that registers only up to 40 pounds of force will not provide a valid measurement because the athlete's strength will likely exceed this range.

Choosing Instruments with Sufficient Sensitivity

For measuring tiny forces, an instrument should be used that can detect these small changes. Otherwise, small changes in the subjects will go unnoticed.

Increasing Items in an Instrument

To increase the power (amount of information) gained with surveys, investigators can use instruments with a larger number of items and a broader scale. For example, using surveys with 40 questions rather than one limited to five questions or using a seven-point scale (ranging from strongly agree to strongly disagree) rather than a two-point scale (agree or disagree)[4] increases the power of an instrument.

Reading the Manual

The manufacturers of measuring instruments often have proprietary information that they may not want to share with consumers. Sometimes researchers have no idea how an instrument works, often referred to as a *black box*. It is important to find out as much as possible about the instrument, formulas used to calculate the data, and generally how to use the equipment properly. For example, some manuals recommend that electronic equipment be warmed up before being operated to achieve stable measurements. The manual also may suggest how frequently to calibrate the equipment.

Calibration of the Measuring Instrument

Calibration is the process of comparing a measuring instrument with some standard.[5] If a scale reads 15 pounds (7 kg) when no weight is loaded, measurements during the study will be incorrect. Calibration is particularly important when the device has been subjected to excessive wear and tear, such as when it is being used by several people.

Triangulation

Use of several methods of data collection can improve the believability and the dimensionality of findings. Results are much more convincing if three different instruments independently suggest the same finding (this is called *triangulation*) than if one tool is used [6] (Figure 18-1).

Accuracy of Software Algorithms or Formulas

It is not safe to assume that software algorithms (formulas) of summary scores such as means and standard deviations are correct. There is always the possibility that there is an error in the formula (a software bug).[7] These formulas are written by human beings. It is good practice to check the accuracy of the output against a known source. That is, check the calculations by hand or from solutions provided in a textbook.

INCONSISTENCIES IN THE SUBJECT

REACTIVITY TO INSTRUMENTS AND TESTING

Subjects may react to measurements. In this problem (called *reactive measures*), measurement affects the thing being measured. Subjects may improve or change their performance over the course of the study because of exposure to the first measurement.[2] Think back to the first time you were tested on something. Did you feel your score was an accurate measure of your true performance? We can learn how to take a test better the

second time around or may relax after being initially self-conscious because we know we are being measured. For example, patients may be self-conscious about being videotaped during gait. Even taking range of motion measurements can affect connective tissue extensibility so that motion at the joint increases on subsequent measure.

In summary, when subjects react to the measuring instrument, investigators may not see a true picture of their performance. This can compromise both internal validity (Was it the treatment or the instrument that caused the change?) and external validity (Would the treatment work in the real world if we had not measured the subjects to death?).

VACCINATION

Posttest Only Control Group Design

Use of a design that lacks a pretest (called a *posttest only control group design*) reduces reactivity and improves the external validity of the study[2,8] (see Chapter 7). With this design, knowledge from a first test (pretest) cannot be used to improve performance on a second test. This is particularly important in a study of attitudes because questions from a pretest can influence responses on subsequent tests.

Practice Sessions

If lack of familiarity is an issue, practice sessions and warm-up trials help subjects become familiar with the setting before measurement.

Passive Measures

Use of passive measures helps reduce reactivity. For example, a one-way mirror can be used rather than a camera placed directly in front of subjects, which may be perceived as too intrusive. For interviews a tape recorder placed inobtrusively in the room may be less reactive than one planted directly in front of a subject.

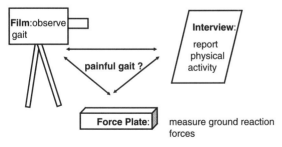

Figure 18-1.   Triangulation, or using multiple methods of data collection, enables a richer interpretation of results. In this example, a painful or antalgic gait may be more fully assessed when kinematic analysis, force plate data, and a questionnaire are included in the analyses.

REFERENCES

1. Carr JJ. *Sensors and Circuits: Sensors, Transducers, and Supporting Circuits for Electronic Instrumentations, Measurement, and Control.* Englewood Cliffs, N.J.: Prentice Hall; 1993.
2. Portney LG, Watkins MP. *Foundations of Clinical Research: Applications to Practice.* Upper Saddle River, N.J.: Prentice Hall; 2000.
3. Hayes KW. Making tests with low reliability work for you. *Orthop Pract.* 1999;11(1):28–29,35.
4. Light RJ, Singer JD, Willett JB. *By Design: Planning Research on Higher Education.* Cambridge, Mass: Harvard University Press, 1990.

5. Johnson SD, Crawford WG. Plane Surveying. In Chen WF, ed. *The Civil Engineering Handbook*. Boca Raton, Fla: CRC Press; 1995:1858–1899.

6. Nachmias CF, Nachmias D. *Research Methods in the Social Sciences*. 5th ed. New York: St. Martin's Press; 1996.

7. Wilkinson L. Task Force on Statistical Inference, APA Board of Scientific Affairs. Statistical methods in psychology journals: guidelines and explanations. *Am Psychol*. 1999;54:594–604.

8. Campbell DT, Stanley JC. *Experimental and Quasi-experimental Designs for Research*. Boston: Houghton Mifflin; 1963.

19

Mistakes in Conducting Studies over Time

Any time a study extends over time (i.e., lasts more than one brief visit) the potential exists for making a number of *temporal* mistakes in research. For example, over time, subjects can become better by learning, growing, developing, healing, or becoming more physically fit, more aware, or wiser. Subjects can become worse over time by becoming bored, less aware, fatigued, sleepy, annoyed, ill, or even die. Any of these effects of time, if unwelcomed, will muddy the results. Guard against them. Temporal problems can be divided into the following three categories (Table 19-1):

1. Changes in the subject's body over time (maturation)
2. Events, news, or gossip over time (history)
3. Departure from the study over time (attrition, mortality)

Table 19-1. Mistakes over Time

Vaccination against Changes within a Subject

- Randomization
- Avoid lifestyle changes
- Design against practice, carry-over, and ordering effects

Vaccination against Events, News, and Gossip

- Be wary of performing longitudinal studies
- Use withdrawal and multiple-baseline designs
- Sample from the same time and geographic area
- Avoid subject cross talk
- Avoid media coverage
- Schedule subjects appropriately
- Conduct an exit interview

Vaccination against Attrition

- Anticipate attrition
- Report the attrition rate
- Analyze the pattern of attrition
- Conduct statistical tests for unequal variance

CHANGES WITHIN THE SUBJECT OVER TIME

From birth through death, the fact is that we grow up and then eventually deteriorate. As we mature we become taller, gain weight, become smarter, become faster, and see better; then the process reverses itself as we age. To a lesser degree, we also may observe changes that occur over the time span of an extended study. The changes that occur within an individual are called *maturation*. They may have nothing to do with the study but can affect the results. A subject can have improvement or deterioration not related to the treatment that therefore should not be attributed to it.

Natural recovery is a good example of a maturational change to guard against in an experiment. H. G. Felsen, a humorist, offered the following observation regarding recovery from the common cold: "Proper treatment will cure a cold in seven days, but left to itself a cold will hang on for a week."[1(p8)]

VACCINATION

Randomization

If groups are compared, randomization can help to distribute subjects who mature at different rates more evenly across the groups. Randomization also can be used to address another threat to internal validity—history (see later).[2]

Avoidance of Lifestyle Changes during the Study

Subjects should be instructed not to engage in new activities that can affect the results because the new activity may be a confounder, for example, adjustments in medications unless medically necessary. A subject who does introduce activities over the course of the study that affect the outcome, may have to be excluded from the study. Otherwise, the change, such as a new medication or a strengthening program, can cause difficulties in interpreting findings. For example, did the strength of subjects 6 through 9 improve because of the treatment or because of the new Jane Smith workout video they used on their own?

Imagine you're determining the effect of a new vitamin on physical endurance and you discover that some of your subjects started going to the gym in the middle of the study. Some of the improvement in endurance from the drug may be the result of the workouts in the gym.

Design against Practice Effects

Repeated testing opportunities can improve performance, not because of a particular intervention but because of a training or practice effect. *Practice makes perfect*. For example, if you are testing golf swing ability, repeatedly measuring golf swing may lead to less error and greater skill. We become better at almost anything we spend more time doing.

If the potential for practice effects is a major concern, a *between-subjects design* can be used so that subjects are not trained through repeated testing. An alternative is to provide subjects with ample practice opportunities until they achieve a stable baseline performance before they are exposed to the treatment.

Design against Carry-over Effects: Between-subjects Design

To test two different treatments, such as different drugs, when the first will aid in performance of the second, a *between-subjects design* (use of separate groups) can be used rather than exposing the same subject to both treatments (within-subject design). Otherwise, the benefit of the first treatment may *carry over* and enhance performance during the second treatment of the same person.

Design against Carry-over Effects: Sufficient Time Intervals between Conditions for Within-subject Designs

Rest periods are needed if carry-over effects are likely in a within-subject design. For studies involving multiple drugs, sufficient time should be allowed for the body to clear (wash out) the effects of the first drug before starting on the second drug.

Fatigue also is a manifestation of a carry-over effect. If the study involves repeated measurements of physical exertion or mental concentration, the subjects should be given rest periods so that fatigue does not become a possible explanation for a subject's deteriorating performance. For example, imagine you are looking at the effects of seven types of music on gait symmetry and notice a trend in which patients adopt a more sluggish, asymmetric gait toward the end of data collection. Can it be that the patients did not have enough rest between trials and are tired? You unwittingly have introduced both music *and fatigue* into the study. The subjects simply did not have enough time to rest, and fatigue carried over to the music conditions. Parenthetically, there is no way to clear, rest, or have a subject forget a learning strategy once learned. In this case, a between-subjects design (described earlier) is appropriate.

Design against Ordering Effects in Within-subject Designs: Use Counterbalance or Crossover Designs

Subjects who receive treatments in a specific order (called *order effect*) may reap an unintended benefit. An example is always providing a heat treatment before an exercise treatment. Persons receiving a heat treatment before exercise may perform better on activities simply because heat precedes the exercise. The heat treatment may improve connective tissue extensibility. Individuals who do not receive heat before exercise may not reap this benefit. Order matters.

To guard against order effects in within-subject designs, each subject should be given treatments in a different order (called *counterbalancing*). If two treatments are involved,[3] a crossover design can be considered, whereby half of the sample received treatment X first followed by treatment Y while the remaining half received treatment Y first followed by treatment X (see Chapter 7). The hope is that with systematic variation of the order of treatments, any potential confounding effect due to sequencing treatment can be spread across all outcomes.

EVENTS, NEWS, AND GOSSIP OVER TIME

The subject may have a special event in life (*history*) that confounds the study and results in a change in performance that is unrelated to the treatment. Some of these confounders include (1) new life strategies, (2) life-altering events, and (3) distracting events.

CONFOUNDING EVENTS

Exposure to New Strategies

A subject may become exposed to a new strategy during a study. For example, a subject who hears that mental imagery improves athletic performance may try imagery in the study to improve his or her performance. The problem is that mental imagery is not an intended treatment (independent variable) in the study and can therefore confound (spoil, corrupt, confuse)[4] the interpretation of a finding.

LIFE-ALTERING EVENTS

Subjects may be exposed to a life-altering event. For example, the responses of a subject being surveyed in 1963 about his or her views of capital punishment may have been affected toward favoring capital punishment by news of the Kennedy assassination. In truth, the subject might not ordinarily have favored capital punishment. The life-altering event, the assassination, therefore affected the subject's score on the survey. Other examples are divorce, financial difficulty, moving, new job, and death or illness in the family. All of these events can indirectly affect subject performance during a study, and the researcher may never know it.

DISTRACTING EVENTS

Subjects may perform poorly because of distraction. For example, student subjects may be scheduled during exam week, when they are preoccupied with grades, are too anxious, or are too tired to focus on an experiment. Another distracter is noise (auditory not statistical) during the experiment.

VACCINATION

Caution with Longitudinal Designs

Longitudinal designs are susceptible to events that occur over time. The longer the study, the more opportunity exists for external events (as well as maturational changes) to introduce themselves into the study. The subject can learn new strategies over time. These effects decrease the internal validity of the results.[3]

Withdrawal and Multiple Baseline Research Designs

To help rule out concerns about history, *time-series designs* (see Chapter 7) can be used. With this method, treatments are withdrawn and readministered, or treatments are staggered (introduced on different days or in different weeks). The idea is that if change in performance follows treatment and does not occur when treatment is not introduced, confounding factors such as external events are more likely to be ruled out as the cause of the change.

Subjects from the Same Time Period

Data from groups should be collected over the same period. Data collected from different eras may compare differently simply because subjects have been exposed to different sets of life experiences at two points in time.[5] For example, subjects' knowledge of and attitudes toward exercise and nutrition in the 1950s may have been different from that of subjects in 2003. It may not be valid to assume groups from different eras are similar in matters related to health and fitness.

Subjects from the Same Geographic Region

Unless a heterogeneous sample is desired to enhance external validity, subjects should be recruited from the same geographic area and have similar life experiences

(history). For example, subjects from urban areas in the United States may walk more quickly than do subjects from rural areas. It may therefore not be valid to assume these groups from different geographic regions are equivalent in matters related to gait.

Avoidance of Cross Talk among Subjects

Subjects should be instructed not to discuss the study with others who are participating in the study so that unique information revealed only to the treatment group is not shared with the control group.[3]

Avoidance of Exposure to Media Coverage

Subjects should be instructed not to seek knowledge about aspects of the study, such as by reading newspapers, searching the Internet, or listening to news reports on television or radio, if such news may influence performance during the study.

Scheduling Subjects

The study should be scheduled so that it is easy for subjects to arrive at the setting without difficulty or fatigue. If it takes a weak patient 2 hours to get to the laboratory during a snowstorm, performance may be negatively affected. Subjects should undergo tests or treatments when the laboratory is least distracting, such as during a quiet time of day or outside exam week.

Exit Interviews

An exit interview should be conducted if there is unexplained improvement in the performance of someone who did not seem likely to improve. The subject might have been privy to biasing information during the study.

ATTRITION

Attrition, also called *experimental mortality,* occurs when subjects leave a study before the study is completed. It does not mean the patient has died, although that is possible. It means the subject chose not to continue in the study. Perhaps the subject was not assigned to the treatment group and therefore did not want to remain in the study. Attrition can affect the results of a study because those who leave the study may have responded differently from those who stay.[2]

Example: Ms. America

Imagine a Ms. America beauty contest in which Ms. New York is clearly the most beautiful and talented contestant but then drops out of the contest in the middle to protest social injustice. Although the runner-up (Ms. Florida) now becomes Ms. America, the outcome does not reflect reality. Ms. New York is still more beautiful and perhaps more ethical, but because she dropped out in the middle of the race, the world will never know it.

VACCINATION

Planning for Attrition

The study should be designed to allow for typical attrition rates. If previous studies suggest a high attrition rate, the options are to increase sample size, choose the population carefully, or keep the study brief.[6] For example, a higher attrition rate can be expected when the subjects are patients with Alzheimer's than when the population is students participating over one semester.

Reporting Attrition Rates

Attrition and response rates (for surveys) should be reported in the results section. Readers can assess the effect of attrition rate only if the rate is reported.[7] Readers need to know how many subjects left the study and why (Is there a pattern?), so they can interpret the results of the study in light of those events.

Analysis of Attrition for Lack of a Random Pattern

Researchers need to identify the reason subjects leave a study. If the reason does not occur in a random pattern, attrition may be related to the study (e.g., the treatment made subjects sick, the task was too difficult; the task was too easy and boring). The result is that unfair comparisons may be made between the two groups.[3] Those who left the study might have improved or diminished group performance scores and provided a more valid finding had they remained in the study.

Statistical Tests

If the variances (variability) in the two groups become unequal because of attrition, a statistical test for unequal variances can be performed.[3]

REFERENCES

1. Huff D. *How to Lie with Statistics.* New York: WW Norton; 1954.
2. Campbell DT, Stanley JC. *Experimental and Quasi-experimental Designs for Research.* Boston: Houghton Mifflin; 1963.
3. Portney LG, Watkins MP. *Foundations of Clinical Research: Applications to Practice.* Upper Saddle River, N.J.: Prentice Hall; 2000.
4. *Webster's New International Dictionary.* 3rd ed., s.v. "confound."
5. Beveridge WIB. *The Art of Scientific Investigation.* 3rd ed. New York: Vintage Books; 1957.
6. Light RJ, Singer JD, Willett JB. *By Design: Planning Research on Higher Education.* Cambridge, Mass: Harvard University Press; 1990.
7. Greenfield MLVH, Kuhn JE, Wojtys EM. A statistics primer: p value—probability and clinical significance. *Am J Sports Med.* 1996;24:863–865.

20

Mistakes in Math

The following data management and statistical issues can influence findings (Table 20-1):

1. Sloppy data entry.
2. Committing Type I and II statistical errors.
3. Violating statistical assumption (using the wrong statistic).

DATA ENTRY ERRORS

VACCINATIONS

Getting Enough Sleep

Researchers should not perform data entry when they are tired, rushed, or jaded. Haste makes waste.

Table 20-1. Mistakes in Math

Vaccination against Data Entry Errors
• Get rest
• Print and recheck entries
• Examine graphs
• Establish procedures for data analysis

Vaccination against Type I Statistical Errors
• Choose an efficient statistical model to analyze data
• Make a statistical adjustment for α level
• Use a strict α level
• Replicate the study

Vaccination against Type II Statistical Errors
• Conduct a power analysis
• Increase the power of the study

Vaccination against Violations of Statistical Assumptions
• Know thy assumptions

Printing and Checking Entries

Entries should be rechecked by the investigator or an uninvolved party. One way to do this is to enter raw data from a logbook into a computer spreadsheet, print the spreadsheet, and then compare, line by line, values between the logbook and the printed spreadsheet.

Examining Graphs: Looking at the Pictures

The raw data should be examined with a scatter plot, histogram, or box plot to identify data that may have been incorrectly entered or included in the analysis. Outliers (extreme values), for example, can dramatically affect the distribution and the statistical findings. Outliers sometimes are caused by simple data-entry errors, such as typing the wrong number in a cell. Statistical software usually has an option for examining outliers in data.[1,2]

Established Procedures for Analyzing Data

It is desirable to use original, raw scores in analysis. Rules for changing raw data, such as transforming or smoothing the data, should be based on established and acceptable procedures so that selected data are not treated preferentially during the analysis. An alternative is to blind the person conducting the analysis from knowledge of the origin of the data so that bias can be minimized. The procedures used to transform data should be described in the results section of the report.

COMMITTING TYPE I AND II ERROR

TYPE I ERROR

Type I error, a false alarm, is finding a significant difference that does not exist. Though the problem of Type I error can always occur due to sampling error, the probability of committing Type I error increases when repeated analyses are conducted on the same set of data. That is, when several hypotheses are tested on the same set of data. Each time a set of data is analyzed, there is a 5% chance that the findings will be significant because of chance. Thus when repeated analyses are conducted, the likelihood increases that results will be found.

VACCINATION

Choosing a Statistic That Allows Efficient Analysis of All the Data

For comparisons of group means, analysis of variance (ANOVA) may be more efficient in testing hypotheses than running several *t* tests, which tend to increase the likelihood of a Type I error.

Statistical Adjustments

The α level can be adjusted if repeated testing is conducted. A Bonferroni correction, a statistical adjustment in which the α level is divided by the number of comparisons, can be used to compensate for the number of repeated analyses (number of comparisons) if several *t* tests are conducted.

Stringent α Level

Setting a conservative α level, such as .01, decreases the power of a test and reduces the risk of a Type I error.

Replication of the Study

Because it is not possible to avoid Type I error with 100% certainty, achieving similar results through replication helps improve confidence in the original findings.[3]

TYPE II ERROR

Type II error, missed opportunity, is not finding a significant difference because the power of the study is too low. Low power often is caused by small sample size. Enrolling more subjects may not be the solution, however. If enough people are tested, it may be possible to detect a small but meaningless effect. For example, with a sufficient sample size, a statistically significant relationship probably can be found between adult shoe size and intelligence. The relationship, however, would be meaningless. If the effect is so small that a huge number of subjects are needed, the study is not worth conducting.

VACCINATION

Power Analysis

The risk of Type II error is minimized through power analysis conducted *before* the study. The results will show how many subjects are needed for the study to detect a statistically significant difference if one really exists.[4]

Increasing the Power

Increased power produces more information and therefore a greater likelihood of detecting statistical significance if differences exist. In general, any procedure that reduces the noise in your data can lead to improved power. The following strategies can help to improve power.

Increasing Sample Size.   Increasing sample size helps to reduce the standard error of the mean and therefore improve the precision of estimating the population mean (see Chapter 11).

Minimization of Attrition.   Loss of subjects reduces the power of a study for the same reason that increasing sample size increases power. As sample size drops, estimates of population values, such as the mean, become less precise.

Use of Parametric Statistics.   Information in a score is fully exploited when parametric statistical tests, such as the Pearson product moment correlation, are conducted. For this reason, continuous data is preferred over categorical data, and normally distributed outcomes are preferred over markedly skewed outcomes so that parametric statistics can be applied.[5]

Use of Higher Measurement Levels.   Lower levels of measurement, such as nominal or categorical, contain less information than higher levels of measurement. As a result, they may not reveal changes in the phenomenon being measured. For example, a good muscle grade is more informative than a score of "within normal limits," and 90 newtons of force is more informative than a good muscle grade. Nominal data should be avoided if ordinal data are available. Ordinal data should be avoided if ratio or interval data are available. The more information in the data, the better the study will be.[5]

Avoidance of Nonparametric Statistics.   Nonparametric analyses, such as Spearman rank correlation, are conducted with ranked data, which contain less information than continuous data.[5]

Use of a Covariate.   The use of covariates in an analysis can improve power by removing a confounding effect on the outcome measure.[5]

Use of Repeated Measures Design.   Repeated measures (within-subject design) are powerful designs because subjects are used as their own controls. This reduces the error (noise) in the measurements because there is little or no variation within each subject.[6]

Reduction in Measurement Error.   Use instruments with acceptable validity and reliability indices. Information is lost when measurements contain error. If measurements are not reliable, a greater sample size may be needed to ensure the same level of statistical power.[5]

Replication of the Study

Repeating the study, perhaps with a more powerful design, that is, using a larger sample size, can reassure investigators about the original findings.[3] This is particularly important when no statistical significance is found in a study that has low power, because other scientists may loose interest in a potentially important topic and move on to more fruitful ground.

VIOLATION OF STATISTICAL ASSUMPTIONS

If a parametric statistical analysis is conducted, assumptions should be checked and satisfied before the analysis is performed. If distributions are not normal, (1) scores have to be transformed to normalize the distribution, (2) nonparametric statistical analysis can be performed if absolutely necessary, or (3) the source of the deviation in the score has to be found. If a measurement or procedural anomaly accounts for the deviation, it may be legitimate to remove the offending points from the study with explanation. An alternative is to analyze the data with and without the unusual cases. This must be documented in the report.

VACCINATION

Common parametric statistical analysis and the associated assumptions follow. Assumption can be tested by means of examining the distributions of each outcome (group of scores) and by performing tests, such as homogeneity of variance, that are commonly included in statistical software packages.

t *Tests*

A *t* test is used for comparisons of two groups.

Assumptions
- *Normal Distribution.* All outcome measures (dependent variables) should have a normal distribution, that is, produce a bell-shaped curve on a graph.
- *Level of Measurement.* Interval or ratio data are required (e.g., 120/80 mm Hg rather than high, normal, and low blood pressure). Ordinal data are used in parametric statistics, although this practice is somewhat controversial.
- *One Measurement of Scores.* Scores are measured only once from each group in independent *t* test analysis. If two scores (related scores) from the same subject are compared (pretest and posttest), a paired (dependent) *t* test is used in the analysis.
- *Similar Group Variability (Homogeneity of Variance).* The scatter or variance (variability in a distribution) in the two groups should be similar. If two

groups differ in variability on an outcome measure, a *t* test for unequal variance can be conducted.

Analysis of Variance

Analysis of variance (ANOVA) is used to compare three or more groups. The assumptions are the same as for a *t* test, and the independent variable (treatment) is at the nominal level (e.g., exercise versus no exercise groups).

Analysis of Covariance

Analysis of covariance (ANCOVA) is used to compare groups with a confounding factor (called a *covariate*) statistically removed or eliminated from the analyses. The assumptions are the same as for ANOVA with the addition of a covariate requirement (the variable to be statistically removed from the analyses). The covariate should

- Be at an interval or ratio level of measurement, not nominal (e.g., number of pounds or kilograms, not obese versus thin).
- Have a linear relationship with the outcome (dependent) variable (e.g., pounds and height).
- Have the same effect on all groups being compared. For example, if caffeine is to be statistically removed, it should affect both men and women or neurology patients and healthy persons to the same degree if these are the groups under study.

Repeated Measures Analysis of Variance

Repeated measures ANOVA is used to compare the effect of all treatments on each subject. The assumptions are the same as for ANOVA with the addition of compound symmetry. The repeated outcomes should be correlated (measures are associated), and the variances (spread of each measure) should be equal across all repeated measures.

Compound symmetry is difficult to satisfy. If this assumption is not met, an ε (epsilon) correction can be used with repeated measured analysis. This value makes the test more conservative.[6]

Multivariate Analysis of Variance

Multivariate analysis of variance (MANOVA) is used to compare groups on more than one outcome. The assumptions are the same as for ANOVA with the addition of the following:

- Scores among all the multiple outcome measures are normally distributed (there is a multivariate normal distribution).
- The correlation between any two dependent variables should be the same in all groups, and the homogeneity of variance assumption for each dependent variable must be satisfied.

Correlational Analysis

Correlational analysis is used to determine the strength of an association between scores on two characteristics.

An example is the Pearson product moment correlation. The requirements are as follows:

- Scores for each characteristic are normally distributed (determined from the histogram).
- Scores for each characteristic have similar variability.
- Scores between the two groups demonstrate a linear (straight-line) relationship on a scatter plot. If the plot is curvilinear, correlational analysis may not be appropriate.

To guard against inappropriate use of correlational analysis, researchers using statistics such as a Pearson product moment correlation need to make sure scores are not restricted within a narrow range, that is, not similar in value. Otherwise, correlations will be underestimated[7] and will not reflect the true association.

For example, when knee range of motion is assessed with two measuring devices, measurements should include a wide range of knee angles (e.g., 0 degrees, 20 degrees, 40 degrees, 60 degrees, 80 degrees, and 120 degrees) rather than only terminal knee extension, the value of which will always be close to 0 degrees.

Regression

Regression is used to establish an equation to make predictions.

- The independent variables should be independent from each other.[8]
- The residual errors should be "well behaved."[8]

There should be a normal distribution of y values (dependent variable) around the regression line (the line with the best accuracy of prediction) for each value of x. This assumption can be evaluated through analysis of the graphs of the residual plots; that is, the difference between the predicted values and the actual values of y.[6]

REFERENCES

1. Loftus G. A picture is worth a thousand p values: on the irrelevance of hypothesis testing in the microcomputer age. *Behav Res Methods Instrum Comput.* 1993;25: 250–256.
2. Wilkinson L. Task Force on Statistical Inference, APA Board of Scientific Affairs. Statistical methods in psychology journals: guidelines and explanations. *Am Psychol.* 1999;54:594–604.
3. Ross LM, Hall BA, Heater SL. Why are occupational therapists not doing more replication research? *Am J Occup Ther.* 1998;52:234–235.
4. Cohen J. *Statistical Power Analysis for the Behavioral Sciences.* 2nd ed. Hillsdale, N.J.: Erlbaum; 1988.
5. Light RJ, Singer JD, Willett JB. *By Design: Planning Research on Higher Education.* Cambridge, Mass: Harvard University Press; 1990.
6. Portney LG, Watkins MP. *Foundations of Clinical Research: Applications to Practice.* Upper Saddle River, N.J.: Prentice Hall; 2000.
7. Welkowitz J, Ewen RB, Cohen J. *Introductory Statistics for the Behavioral Sciences.* 5th ed. Fort Worth, Tex: Harcourt Brace College; 1998.
8. Schroeder LD, Sjoquist DL, Stephan PE. *Understanding Regression Analysis: An Introductory Guide.* Newbury Park, Calif: Sage Publications; 1986.

Part IV
The Examination

21

Evaluating Research: Is It Believable?

GOAL OF A CRITIQUE

The goal of reading a research report is to decide for yourself whether the author's newly acquired knowledge is believable. Weighing all aspects of a study fairly and without being too exacting on small issues, do you believe the outcome of the study? Because any one study can be wrong due to sampling error alone, that is, through chance, *replication is important*.

The evaluation is divided into three main sections using the metaphor of a play in three acts (Tables 21-1 through 21-3). Within each *act*, questions are raised that may affect the internal and external validity of the report. Refer to Parts II and III of this book for a review of fundamental concepts and a discussion of internal and external validity.

ACT I: THE BEGINNING

TITLE

Critique Question

- Does the title broadcast the true nature of the study?

The title of the report should give the reader a clear idea of the question that will be investigated. Words in the title such as *effects of, influence,* or *affect* suggest causality,[1] whereas the word *relationship* indicates an association. The title should clearly represent the intent of the report.

Examples of Titles
- The Effects (or Influence) (or Impact) of Kryptonite on Superpower [causality]
- Is Kryptonite Related to Superpower? [association]

The Information in a Title

Unlike the title of a film on a marquee of a theater, such as *Rocky* or *Superman,* the title of a research study must include additional information, such as the independent and

Table 21-1. Act I: The Introduction

Section	Purpose
Title	Convey intent of article
Key words	Provide search words for computer
Authors	Show expertise, authorities, biases
Abstract	Summarize study
Problem	Identify research area
Background	Describe what has been done
Question	Convey the specific purpose
Theory	Discuss possible explanations
Hypothesis	Make a prediction based on possible explanation
Statistical analysis	Explain how data were analyzed

dependent variables. A film title would read *Superman.* The title of a research report, however, would read "The Effect of Kryptonite on the Flying Ability of Supermen." Included are the independent variable (kryptonite), the dependent variable (flying ability), and the population (supermen). Extra words, such as "A Study of" are superfluous.[2]

KEY WORDS

Words such as *clinical trial* in a title can help the reader conduct a literature search to find the article.[3]

AUTHORS

Critique Questions

- Are authors authorities on the research topic?
- Do authors have a known bias, pet theory, or subscribe to a school of thought?

The names and credentials of the investigators who write a report can be informative. Well-known investigators in a field of study are often viewed as the authorities.

129

Investigators with a research degree such as a doctorate are expected to be adequately versed in design and analysis. Graduate students, whose scholarship may be considerable, can make important contributions to the literature. By convention, the first author listed usually is the one who has contributed most to the work. The contribution of the other authors is less clear and may be substantially less than that of the first author.[4]

Identify any personal biases in the authors if possible,[3] especially in qualitative studies in which the author is actively engaged with subjects during data collection. Sometimes an author's theoretical viewpoint can be determined by means of reading his or her past publications.

ABSTRACT

Critique Question

- Is the abstract limited only to findings contained within the report? You may need to read the study and then reread the abstract to answer this question.

The abstract (a brief synopsis of the study) enables the reader to decide whether the subject matter is of great enough interest to read further. The information in the abstract may indicate the target audience and therefore the readers who may best use the findings from the study. Like a billboard in front of a playhouse, the abstract summarizes the "plot" of the report (the problem, the setting, the actors, the conflict and resolution). The content of the abstract, which is generally limited to 300 words or fewer[3] typically includes background, purpose, method, analysis, results, discussion, and conclusions.

One red herring to watch out for in the abstract is claims of findings that are either omitted or inconsistently reported in the body of the article. One study found 18% to 68% of the abstracts in several prestigious medical journals to be deficient.[5] The abstract often is the first and sometimes is the only thing a reviewer reads when investigators are seeking funding or publication. For this reason, it is important that it clearly reflect the body of the report.

INTRODUCTION

The introduction is the beginning portion of the research's story. It includes the general problem area, the literature review, the specific question, the hypothesis (prediction or tentative answer), and the rationale for the hypothesis (the theory).

THE PROBLEM

Critique Question

- Is the overall problem clinically important enough to address?

The problem usually is the bigger issue ("the forest") from which the author will try to whittle down to a more manageable question ("the tree") in the study. Problems tend to shock, horrify, or at least wake up the reader to the importance of the study. Statistics often are used to support a point. For example, authors may state that more than x million persons in the United States have Parkinson's disease or that cancer is the number one killer in the United States. These statements reduce the chance that a reader will say, "So what?" "This research is not important enough for me to read," instead "If x million people have Parkinson's disease or if cancer is the number one killer, it's obvious that you've got my attention."

BACKGROUND (LITERATURE REVIEW)

Critique Questions

- Is there adequate coverage to sense the full scope of the problem?
- Are important journal citations omitted, leading to a biased review?

The literature review gives the reader a sense of the current state of knowledge on the problem. Authors frequently review relevant studies, critique previous studies that have weaknesses, and identify current theories that may explain the problem. A dearth of studies or a controversy gives the investigator justification to embark on a new study by stating that "few studies have been done in this area" or that "two competing theories have been proposed to explain the phenomenon." Older literature, although valid at the time of publication, may no longer be relevant by today's standards. For example, fitness outcomes in the past may have been different if subjects in the past had had modern diet and exercise information available to them.[6]

Comments

Be Current. The literature review should be current, the sources sufficient in number, and citations published within the past 5 to 10 years. Literature older than 10 years may be considered of historical value only.[3] A few classic (old and important) articles are useful to place the study in historical perspective. If there is no recent literature on the subject, the author should state so (e.g., "An exhaustive literature review failed to reveal . . ."). The average number of references is 28.[3]

Be Complete. All relevant reports should be cited. Original thinkers also need to be credited. An author who reports developing a novel method of assessment may not in fact be the first. Angry letters to the editor from the originator may be published to set the record straight.[7,8]

Be Scholarly. Critiques of the literature should have a scholarly tone. Previous studies should not be condemned because of professional jealousy or political motive. On more than one occasion, I have heard of studies being unjustifiably dismissed because the reviewer's own research was not cited.

THE QUESTIONS (PROBLEM STATEMENT, RESEARCH QUESTIONS)

Critique Question

- Is the question important enough to escape the "so what?" reaction from readers.

The Trilogy

The right question has three requirements[6]—feasibility, importance, and answerability. It is in the introduction that the reader can pose the question "so what?" if the author's question does not seem to be clinically important.

Completeness

The question should include the group (population) under study, the variables, and what the author seeks to accomplish (e.g., a description, a relationship, a treatment effect).

Examples of Problem Statements: Superman
- To describe the superpowers of speed, strength, and flying ability among supermen.
- To determine whether there is a positive relationship between cape length and flying ability among supermen.
- To determine the effect of kryptonite on speed, strength, and flying ability among supermen.

Examples of Problem Statements: Parkinson's Disease
- To describe motor deficits among patients with second-stage Parkinson's disease.
- To determine whether a relationship exists between hand tremor and stress level among patients with second-stage Parkinson's disease.
- To determine the effect of rhythmical music on the gait symmetry among patients with second-stage Parkinson's disease.

Are Variables Adequately Defined?

Authors need to define operationally all the variables so that readers know exactly what is meant by each variable (and how they are measured) such as speed (Is it average velocity or instantaneous velocity?), strength (Is it a manual muscle test, power, isometric, or torque?), or flying ability (Is it distance covered or height of flight?).

Is Replication the Goal?

Do the authors want to replicate previous studies (perhaps using a different setting or age group) to further enhance ability to generalize findings to a population? No one study can prove a finding because results can always be attributed to sampling error (chance). Replication is the rule in science.

THEORY

Critique Question

- Is the research driven or guided by theory?

If the authors discuss theory, the research is considered theory based and typically includes a hypothesis to allow a prediction based on the theory. If there is no theory, why not? Are the authors simply interested in evaluating the outcome of an intervention (the what) rather than going deeper to understand the mechanism (the how) behind the outcome?

HYPOTHESIS

Critique Questions

- Are hypotheses stated?

Hypotheses are part of a deductive form of reasoning and should be stated if the authors suggest a theory. For example, "If gravity is operating whereby things accelerate at a rate of 9.8 m/s^2, then the apple in my study also should accelerate toward the ground at that same rate."

- Are hypotheses stated before data collection is described?

If the authors state a hypothesis, it should be clear that they did so *before* data collection was conducted. (You can't place your bets once the horses have finished the race.)[9]

- Do hypotheses clearly predict a relationship?

Are hypotheses clearly stated? The hypotheses should clearly indicate the predicted relationship between the independent and dependent variables.

- Is there a sufficient number of hypotheses?

There should be a sufficient number of separate hypotheses to answer the question. A separate hypothesis for interactions, if examined, should be included.

- Can each hypothesis be rejected or accepted?

A hypothesis can be supported or rejected. It cannot be partially rejected. You cannot be partially pregnant, and your hypothesis similarly cannot be partially correct. If all components of a question are included in one huge hypothesis (not a good idea), and if only one portion of this hypothesis is rejected because of the findings, the whole hypothesis must be rejected.

Example

There will be a positive relationship between lung cancer and secondhand smoke among young and elderly adults.

In the example above, to reject the hypothesis, all relationships in the prediction must be satisfied. It would be wise to separate the hypotheses by age group. That is, present separate hypotheses for young and elderly adults.

STATISTICAL ANALYSIS

Critique Question

- Are statistical analyses appropriate for the design and the type of data collected in the study?

A logical choice of analysis should be based on the question and the design (see Chapter 13). The type of data also helps determine the analysis performed. Nominal (categorical) data require nonparametric statistics. Information at the interval and ratio levels of measurement can best be exploited through parametric statistics. There should be a sufficient number of analyses to test the different hypotheses.

Example

A question that seeks to describe the characteristics of one person may be answered with a descriptive design, such as case report, and descriptive statistics, using measures of central tendency such as the mean; measures of dispersion such as standard deviation; percentages; or absolute error.

A question that seeks to examine the relationship between age and gait velocity can be answered with a correlational design to relate the two variables and perhaps a Pearson correlation statistical analysis to provide an index of how strongly the two variables vary together.

A question that seeks to examine the effect of a treatment on three groups of patients can be answered with a single-factor between-subjects design and analysis of variance (ANOVA).

Is an α Level Stated?

The α level, the maximal risk of falsely reporting a finding, should be established *before* data collection is conducted.[3,9]

Is the Statistical Package Mentioned?

The statistical software package should be described (e.g., SPSS and the version) so that others can use similar methods of analysis to replicate the findings.

ACT II: THE METHOD

The methods section, which is probably the most important part of a report, often is glossed over or even skipped by readers.[10] The method has enormous bearing on the believability (internal and external validity) of a study because it tells the reader what was done during the experiment or observation (Table 21-2). A reader who skips the methods section assumes that the authors executed a perfect study. This is rarely the case. The methods section often has shortcomings. *Don't skip it.*

Table 21-2. Act II: The Method

Component	What to Ask
Design	Is it an experiment or an observation (nonexperiment)?
Sample	
Composition	Is the population relevant to practice?
Selection	Is the sample representative?
Number	Is a power analysis reported?
Setting	Is the setting appropriate?
Instruments	Are validity and reliability reported?
Procedures	Are they clear, relevant, and consistent?

THE DESIGN

Is the Design Clearly Stated?

Critique Questions

- If a description or association is sought, is an appropriate nonexperimental design used?
- If a cause-and-effect relationship is sought, is an appropriate experimental design used?

The authors should clearly state their research design and the independent and dependent variables. The design should not be withheld or disguised to keep the reader guessing, as in a murder mystery. Readers should avoid disparaging a design simply because it is not their favorite one.[11] Every design (even your own) possesses strengths and weaknesses. The key is whether the design helps to answer the question.

Example of a Clearly Stated Design

"A single factor, between-subjects design was employed in this study. Spinach was the independent variable, and strength was the dependent variable."

Can the Design Answer the Question?

Nonexperimental Design. If the study is exploratory and the investigators seek to describe, a descriptive design is all that is needed because causality is not a concern. If the investigator seeks to examine associations, a correlational design is needed because causality is not an issue. For a valid (believable) conclusion, all descriptive studies still require a representative sample, unbiased investigators, and objective, valid measures. Correlational designs require appropriate statistical analysis.

Experimental Design. If the investigator seeks to examine causality, an experimental or quasiexperimental design is needed because a study with strong internal validity is critical to demonstrating causality. Consider the following list to evaluate true experimental and quasiexperimental designs when the investigator wants to demonstrate a causal relationship (see Chapters 15 through 20).

COMPARISON GROUPS.   Does the design include a comparison group to enhance internal validity?

RANDOMIZATION.   Does the design control or minimize the affects of extraneous factors? Random assignment is the preferred method of controlling extraneous factors in experiments. Random assignment helps secure equivalence across groups before a treatment is introduced to one of them. Intact groups may not be equivalent, and internal validity may be compromised.

When randomization is not feasible, other methods of measuring and adjusting for potential confounding factors, either through analysis with covariates or designs using matching or blocking, should be considered.[11]

MANIPULATION OF THE INDEPENDENT VARIABLE.   Are the treatments (independent variable) sufficiently manipulated so that they clearly occur before and therefore are capable of having a causal effect on the outcome measures?

EXAMINATION OF INTERACTIONS.   Are interaction effects examined to enhance the external validity (real-life application) of the study. That is, has a two-way factorial design been used?

REACTIVITY.   Is a posttest only control group design used to guard against cofounders during testing if subjects are reactive to measurements? Such a situation may arise when the subjects' exposure to a pretest influences or cues performance on the posttest.

CONFOUNDING EFFECTS OF TIME.   If studies stretch out over time, are procedures in place to guard against problems of history (special knowledge), maturation (growth, healing, learning), or attrition (dropping out of the study)?

ADDRESS PRACTICE AND LEARNING EFFECTS.   Is a between-subject design used to guard against confounders such as learning or practice?

ORDERING EFFECTS.   Is a counterbalanced (crossover) design instituted to guard against ordering effects in within-subject (repeated measures) designs.

SAMPLE AND POPULATION: WHO?

Critique Questions

- From what population has the author taken the sample?
- Is this population important to your research or clinical practice?

How Much Variability Is There in the Sample?

Is the sample homogeneous or heterogeneous? A homogeneous sample with clearly defined inclusion criterion improves internal validity. A heterogeneous sample improves the ability to generalize the findings, or external validity, of the study at the expense of internal validity.[6]

What Are the Inclusion and Exclusion Criteria?

The characteristics of the population under study largely determine how the findings can be applied and interpreted.[11] For example, findings among active healthy elderly adults may not be generalized to physically inactive persons and residents of nursing homes.

Subject Incentives

Have the subjects been promised money or other compensation for their participation, suggesting that the sample recruited may not be typical of the average person from that population? Use of compensation can limit external validity. Subjects who have selected themselves because of financial considerations may be different from those who are more altruistic or less concerned with compensation.

Who Screens the Potential Subjects?

Is the person conducting the screening qualified to do so, such as a physician, physical therapist, occupational therapist, or psychologist, depending on the type of assessment?

Does the Group Have Extreme Scores?

If the sample consists of groups of individuals with extreme scores, regression toward the mean may occur and compromise internal validity.

Has the Hawthorne Effect Occurred?

Subjects' knowledge of their participation in a study can influence their behavior.[12]

SAMPLING: WHAT METHOD?

Critique Question

- Do sampling procedures assemble a representative sample from the population so that reasonable generalizations to the population can be made?

The sampling method must be clearly stated. Random selection (probability sampling) better reflects the population to which the authors want to generalize findings. A convenience sample may limit generalization. Readers may question the objectivity of an author who conceals the use of convenience sampling.[11] Results with this nonprobability sampling method cannot be generalized to a larger population and are limited to the sample described and to persons with the same characteristics.[13]

SAMPLE SIZE: HOW MANY?

Critique Questions

- Is the sample size so large that anyone could find a statistically significant result?
- Is the sample size so small that no one could find a statistically significant result?

- Was a power analysis conducted to determine a sample size sufficient to find a statistically significant and important result if one exists?

How was the sample size justified? Power analysis? Pilot study? The literature? Or was there no rationale for sample size, that is, was a number pulled out of thin air? Power analysis is currently the accepted way of determining sample size for a study and should be included in the report.[11] For example, the investigator may state "a sample size of 64 was determined, based on a power of .80, and α level of .05, and a moderate effect size of .50."

In general, at least 30 subjects in a sample are necessary to estimate the population characteristics.[13] Small samples tend to have greater variability in their scores and do not reflect the population. Use of a small sample also may increase the probability of Type II error (missing a finding). Use of an excessively large sample, however, may lead to an overly expensive study and a statistically significant difference that is not necessarily important (Type I error).[14]

SETTING: WHERE?

Critique Questions

- Is the setting experimentally controlled enough to ensure internal validity if a cause-and-effect relationship is being sought?
- Is the setting real enough or relevant to your practice to ensure external validity?
- Is the study conducted in an artificial (laboratory) or a more natural setting?

A controlled, artificial setting improves the internal validity of a study, whereas a more natural setting enhances external validity. A multicenter study with many geographic locations may have less internal validity (lack of control over history) but more external validity (efficacy demonstrated at multiple sites).

ETHICAL ISSUES

Use of Human Subjects in Research

In research with human beings, ethical standards must be upheld to ensure the subjects' rights are protected. There also are rules for research with animals. The ethical standards are necessary because there can be a conflict between the researcher's desire to help patients and a desire to advance scientific knowledge.[15]

Guidelines for conducting research on human subjects[16] were developed and revised by the World Medical Association after World War II[17] and are contained in the Declaration of Helsinki.[18] The basic principles are as follows:

- The study must conform to scientific principles and knowledge of the scientific literature.

- Experimental procedures must be reviewed by a specially appointed committee.
- Qualified persons must conduct the research.
- The importance of the study must be proportional to the risks to the subjects.
- Benefits to the subjects and others must be weighed against the risks.
- The rights and privacy of the subjects must be safeguarded.
- Results must be accurately reported.
- Subjects must be informed of aims, methods, anticipated benefits, potential hazards and discomforts during the study, and their freedom to abstain and withdraw consent to participate at any time without penalty.
- Subjects must be able to consent freely, preferably in writing, without duress.
- If a subject is legally incompetent, consent must be obtained from a legal guardian in accordance with national legislation. When incapacity (mental, physical, being a minor) makes consent impossible, consent must be obtained from a responsible relative in accordance with national legislation. If a minor is able to give consent, consent must be obtained from both the minor and the legal guardian.

The protocol should contain a statement of compliance with ethical principles.

Institutional Review Board.   Have the procedures of the study been reviewed by an institutional review board (IRB)? IRBs are designated to interpret the ethical guidelines and review research proposals to determine whether researchers comply with the principles. The IRB is interested in what researchers will ask patients *to do* in a study and in evaluating studies for scientific merit.[18] IRBs are not necessarily interested in research ideas. Most journals require a statement regarding IRB approval before a report can be considered for publication.

Informed Consent.   Have the subjects been informed they are in a study and did they sign a consent form that they have agreed to participate? A consent form informs subjects of their *rights* and *what is going to be done* to them. Subjects sign such a form *before* enrolling in a study. Although they sign consent forms, subjects may not understand their rights in a study.[19] Any potential conflict of interest between the authors and subjects whereby subjects may feel required to participate, such as clinician–patient or professor–student relationships, should be disclosed.

KNOWLEDGE OF THE HYPOTHESIS.   Knowledge of the investigator's hypothesis (bias), if it is unintentionally included in the informed consent, can influence subjects' performance. This may be difficult to assess without access to the consent form.

Treatment of Subjects.   How should subjects be treated? The answer is, the way you would like yourself or your own family to be treated. Charlie Sprague, Director of Research Development, NYU School of Education, offers good advice for working with human subjects: "Put yourself in their shoes."

INSTRUMENTATION

Identification of the Instrument

Are the measuring instruments described sufficiently (model number, name and location of manufacturer) so that the study can be replicated using the same equipment?[11]

Properties of the Instrument

Are instrument characteristics described (range, threshold, sensitivity, accuracy, precision) so that the reader can evaluate the appropriateness of the instruments used in the study? A picture of the instrument (experimental setup) is helpful to readers.

Validity and Reliability

Are validity and reliability of all measuring instruments reported? Simply stating that validity and reliability was acceptable, without providing indices (e.g., r, ICC) is unacceptable.

Are validity and reliability pertinent to scores of the population under study,[11] documented through pilot work, or determined during the study to enhance the credibility of the findings? Are the reliability coefficients high enough, that is, greater than the .90 recommended for clinical measures?[6] Hayes[20] suggests that for adequate clinical decision making, reliability of continuous data should exceed .80 and of categorical data, .70 (see Chapter 9).

Invasiveness of the Instrument

Are measures invasive? Invasive or artificial measures, such as needle sticks, may cause subjects to be reactive (respond in ways they would not normally) and compromise the external validity of the study.

Is Triangulation Incorporated into the Design?

Multiple methods of measurement (triangulation) can provide rich, convincing dimensionality to the dependent variable.

PROCEDURES

Critique Questions

- Are the treatment procedures relevant to your research interests or clinical practice?
- Are procedures standardized to enhance the internal validity of an experiment?
- Are procedures clear enough to allow replication by others?

Are the Procedures or Treatments Clearly Described?

The procedures should be clear enough for anyone to replicate if necessary. Are the treatments (independent variables) operationally defined in the study so that the reader can determine whether the findings can be generalized to interventions employed in the clinic? Tightly controlled conditions enhance internal validity. More naturalistic conditions enhance external validity.

Blinding

What safeguards are in place to protect against experimental bias? Simply acknowledging awareness of investigator bias (i.e., "I am aware of my hypothesis and am therefore resolved to remain objective.") does not magically remove the investigator's hand from influencing the outcome. Double-blind procedures should be instituted if the opportunity arises.[11]

Are Procedures Standardized?

Standardized procedures for administering treatments (independent variable) and taking measurements (dependent variable) help ensure a consistent environment for all subjects. For example, instructions can be tape-recorded or read from a script. Procedures that are not standardized may do the opposite. A checklist can help ensure that steps in the procedures are not skipped.

Who Administered the Intervention?

Are treatments administered by "real" clinicians, or were treatments administered by a specialist outside the field with special knowledge? The former enhances external validity, and the latter limits external validity to only those specialists.

ACT III: RESULTS

THE ORDER OF REPORTING FINDINGS

Critique Questions

- Before hypothesis testing, were statistical assumptions checked and satisfied (are dependent variables normally distributed)?
- Do the results seem plausible from an examination of the means, standard deviations, and graphs of the distributions?
- Are the results statistically significant, indicating that findings are reliable and probably not due to chance?
- Is the magnitude of change (effect size) impressive in terms of your research interests or clinical practice?

Unforeseen Complications in the Study.   Were complications and unexpected events reported? Just as you would report a hurricane that ruined your fishing trip before

Table 21-3. Act III: Results

Component	What to Ask
Results	
Complications	Any attrition or outliers?
Descriptives	Are distributions normal?
Statistical	Are assumptions satisfied?
assumptions	
Inferentials	
Hypothesis testing	Are null hypotheses rejected?
Power	Was study sensitive enough to detect real differences?
Effect size	Is the magnitude of any change clinically impressive?
Figures and tables	Are they clear? Do they reflect the truth?
Discussion	Are the findings reflected on and interpreted?
Confirm theory	What is the mechanism?
Compare and contrast	Is there support from other studies?
Limitations	Are any potential biases or limitations discussed?
Clinical implications	Are the findings important to patient care?
Future	Is another study suggested?
Conclusion	Are the primary findings reported?
References and	Are primary sources used? Are the references current?
acknowledgments	
Tone	Is the tone scholarly or emotional?
Intelligibility	Is the article readable? Does the author sidestep the facts?
Footnotes	What are the funding sources? Are there conflicts of interest?

describing your catch, you also should report unplanned problems with the study before outcomes are reported.[11] Complications may include lack of response, missing data, outliers (extreme scores), and attrition (loss of subjects), all of which can result in an undesirably nonrepresentative sample pool. Nonrandom attrition, where a pattern is found, is troublesome and can lead to a bias in the remaining sample. If any of the subjects drop out of the study, there should be an attempt to uncover the reason.

Descriptives

Each dependent variable (outcome) should first be individually described in terms of its central tendency, variability, symmetry, and outliers. Combined, this information describes the basic properties of the variable.

Statistical Assumptions

Are all dependent variables normally distributed? If statistical assumptions for data are not checked and satisfied or reported, it is impossible to determine whether results

of the statistical tests are valid. Did the authors transform the raw scores to normalize a skewed distribution before applying parametric statistics? Parametric analysis may be inappropriate if statistical assumptions regarding the results (e.g., a severely skewed distribution) are violated.

Inferential Statistics

Descriptive statistics should be followed by tests of significance. Reporting in the reverse order (inferential before descriptive statistics) is like seeing the end of a movie before the beginning.

Testing the Hypotheses. Are the hypotheses restated and either rejected or not rejected on the basis of the results of the statistical analysis? Authors should be informative about the results. It is more informative to specify a specific P value (e.g., $P = .02$) than to simply state that the null hypothesis was rejected or that the P value is less than .05. *Confidence intervals* can give the reader additional information about the location of the mean score of a performance for a given population.[11]

Reporting Power

If the findings are not significant, do the authors report results of a power analysis to determine whether power was too low (insensitive) to detect a significant difference that may have been present. That is, was a Type II error likely? The power of a study can be determined using power tables once sample size, α level, and *actual* effect size are provided.

Reporting Effect Size

Are effect sizes (the magnitude of effect or strength of a treatment) reported so that readers can determine whether the results were clinically important? Clinical importance often is a judgment.[21] An effect size can be as meaningful as a nonstandardized mean difference (e.g., number of cigarettes smoked per day) or can be in standardized units, such as a correlation coefficient (r).[11] The following indices, which are sometimes reported, can be used as a rough guide for the effect of treatment[22]:

- A small effect size is too small to see with the naked eye (index = .20).
- A medium effect size is large enough to see with the naked eye (index = .50).
- A large effect size is grossly observable (index = .80).

Tables and Figures

Tables and figures both are useful because readers may process information more easily using either one of the formats.[11] Tables provide detailed information whereas figures can illustrate the pattern of the data effectively. The question is, are they understandable? Do figures have clearly marked legends on the x and y axes? Are the axes nearly equal in length, or are they grossly distorted (e.g., one axis twice the length of the other).[23] The reader should not have to waste 10 minutes deciphering an author's graphs.

Other Statistical Concerns

Confirmed Equivalence of Groups. Did the authors confirm group equivalence in an experiment? If groups were not equivalent, was a statistical adjustment such as analysis of covariance (ANCOVA) performed to make the groups equivalent on the pretest and to enhance the internal validity of the experiment?

Conducting Repeated Analyses: Beating a Dead Horse. Were unnecessary repeated analyses performed on the same set of data, thus increasing the likelihood of Type I error (finding significance where there isn't any)? This often is a problem when repeated *t* tests are conducted without a conservative corrective procedure such as a Bonferroni correction.[24]

Supplementary Analysis

A supplementary section gives the researcher an opportunity to examine other relationships and group differences that were not part of the original purpose of the report, that is, those not hypothesized. Any post hoc analysis should be used to generate new hypotheses rather than to test them.[2] Interesting findings unearthed from supplementary analysis can then serve as a focal point in future confirmatory studies.

DISCUSSION

Critique Questions

- Do the authors make sense of the data and interpret them in terms of theory?
- Do the authors attempt to build on the work of previous findings?
- Are potential biases or limitations in the study discussed?

The purpose of the discussion is to reflect on the data and make sense of them. The discussion section of a report is not necessarily the truth of the study but is the author's interpretation of the findings. The reader need to consider whether the results of the study seem credible or incredible on the basis of theory and outcomes of previous studies.[11]

INDUCTIVE REASONING

Inductive reasoning, that is, making inferences from the data,[2] often is incorporated into the discussion section of a report (Figure 21-1). Given the data collected, what can we now say about the theory (e.g., "The wind tunnel data from this study appear to confirm Mary Poppins' theory of air travel.")? Authors developing theory may reflect on their data (evidence) and search for any patterns that

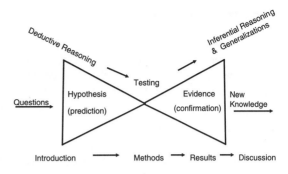

Figure 21-1. Deductive and inductive thinking in a report.

emerge and can be developed into a principle. It is the beginning of theory development.

DO THE DATA FIT THE THEORY?

If they are testing a theory, the authors may state how the data from the study either confirm or disconfirm the theory. If it is not disconfirmed (a strange but proper term), the theory remains a viable explanation for the phenomenon under study. The data still fit the theory.

BUILDING ON THE KNOWLEDGE BASE OF OTHERS

Do findings connect with those of previous studies? Investigators should use new findings to build on the findings of others so that knowledge base can grow. Do the findings corroborate or disagree with previous findings? Comparing the effect size with those of previously published studies allows readers to assess the stability (consistency) of the results across different conditions cited in the literature.[11] Discrepancies with other studies should be explored in terms of differences in methods, such as using a different instrument; differences in sampling design, such as using a convenience sample with healthy young subjects; differences in analysis, such as using a less powerful, nonparametric statistic; and differences in theoretical interpretations.

ARE BIASES AND LIMITATIONS IN THE STUDY DISCUSSED?

There are no perfect studies. The authors should indicate any important weaknesses or limitations in their own study that would tend to compromise internal validity. Although the authors need not bare their souls to the scientific community, important threats to validity—icebergs that sink the research boat—should be disclosed so that readers can fairly assess the study.[25] The authors also should indicate any limitations in the design that would limit the ability to generalize their findings to a larger population (external validity).

ARE THERE CONNECTIONS TO CLINICAL PRACTICE?

Most important and frequently missing, do the authors connect their findings to clinical practice?[3] Is the effect of the treatment impressive enough to warrant use by the clinicians?

FOLLOW-UP STUDY

Do the authors recommend how the knowledge base can be further developed? Have they recommend thoughtful follow-up studies?[3,11]

CONCLUSION

Critique Question

- Do the authors confine their concluding remarks to the primary findings of the study or do they celebrate an unrelated finding that has no bearing on the original intent of the research?

RESEARCH AS A WORKING PAPER

It is critical that the authors conclude only what they find objectively in their study and no more. One study rarely can prove a phenomenon because mistakes and unavoidable errors (sampling error, Type I and Type II errors) are always possible. A study should be considered a working paper that contributes by adding another piece to the puzzle. Conclusions should be viewed as tentative until a body of evidence accumulates.[26]

THE FINAL WORD

At the end of the report, you should draw your own conclusions about the credibility of the study.[27]

REFERENCES

Critique Questions

- Are references current, accurately recorded, and sufficient in number for what is known about the topic?
- Are references from secondary sources (filtered or watered down), thus casting a shadow on the trustworthiness of these sources?

Sloppy, incomplete, or inaccurate references may suggest other problems with the report; that is, they may be the tip of the iceberg. Primary sources such as research reports provide direct information from authors who had intimate contact with the data.[28] Secondary sources such as textbooks and review articles may contain filtered information (Figure 21-2).

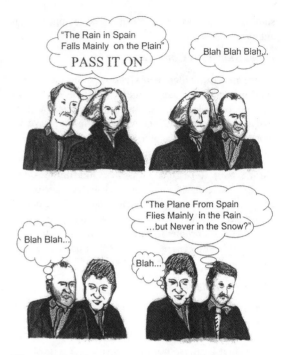

Figure 21-2. Secondary sources. Much like the game telephone, secondary sources such as books, review articles, and reports from the news media can filter and sometimes distort the communications of findings.

Imagine the game telephone whereby the first person (a primary source) whispers information to the second person. The message is passed sequentially through dozens of ears until it gets to a 30th person (the reader). By the time the message is transmitted from the first to the last person, the information may be watered down or completely inaccurate.

MISCELLANEOUS FACTORS

TONE OF THE REPORT

Critique Question

- Does the tone of the report appeal to the reader's emotions rather than reason, suggesting a lack of objective evidence on which to base the conclusions?

Readers often can sense the author's tone in a report. The tone should be commensurate with the quality of the research and always should be scholarly (knowledge seeking) in nature. Unjustified arrogance, such as "I have proved for the first time," should be evaluated cautiously.[25] A scholarly approach is always appreciated. For a good example of humble giants, read Watson and Crick's 1953 proposal for the structure of DNA: "It has not escaped our notice that the specific pairing we have postulated immediately suggests a possible copying mechanism for the genetic material."[29]

ACKNOWLEDGMENTS

It usually is impossible to conduct research without the help of others. Those contributions should be acknowledged. Watson and Crick acknowledged three colleagues, their coworkers, and one foundation.[29]

READABILITY

Critique Question

- Is the report unintelligible, suggesting the author may be trying to equivocate, or sidestep the facts?

The readability of a report is the responsibility of the author.[25] Jargon, which does not clearly communicate ideas, can alienate readers such as clinicians.[30] There is, unfortunately, a positive association between unintelligible research writing and prestige. The less understandable the writing, the more we tend to admire the writer ($r = .70$).[31] Perhaps the reason for much of the clouded prose is to protect oneself from criticism.[32] If the author does not take a stand, how can he or she be criticized? To some, the motto unfortunately has been: "If you can't convince them, confuse them."[31]

FOOTNOTES

Critique Question

- Does the presence of a corporate funding source, such as a drug company, suggest a conflict of interest or bias in the study?

It often is instructive to read the footnotes, which can reveal who funded the study. Readers need to be leery of studies funded by or conducted within an industry, such as by a pharmaceutical company that stands to make a profit on favorable findings. Independent replication of the first study may be indicated if bias due to conflict of interest exists.

REFERENCES

1. Halperin S. Spurious correlations: causes and cures. *Psychoneuroendocrinology.* 1986;11:3–13.
2. Iverson C, Flanagin A, Fontanarosa PB, et al. *American Medical Association Manual of Style.* 9th ed. Baltimore: Williams & Wilkins; 1998.
3. Braddom CL. A framework for writing and/or evaluating research papers. *Am J Phys Med Rehabil.* 1990;69:333–335.
4. Shapiro DW, Wenger NS, Shapiro MF. The contributions of authors to multiauthored biomedical research papers. *JAMA.* 1994;271:438–442.
5. Pitken RM, Branagan MA, Burmeister LF. Accuracy of data in abstracts of published research articles. *JAMA.* 1999;281:1110–1111.
6. Portney LG, Watkins MP. *Foundations of Clinical Research: Applications to Practice.* Upper Saddle River, N.J.: Prentice Hall; 2000.
7. Owens DF Jr. A new technique of tissue stiffness (compliance) assessment: Its reliability, accuracy, and comparison with an existing method [Letter]. *J Manipulative Physiol Ther.* 1996;19:357.
8. Herzog W. In reply. *J Manipulative Physiol Ther.* 1996;19:358.
9. Bailar JC III. Science, statistics, and deception. *Ann Intern Med.* 1986;104:259–260.
10. Fitzgerald FT. From Galen to Xerox: the authoritarian reference in medicine. *Ann Intern Med.* 1982;96:245–246.
11. Wilkinson L. Task Force on Statistical Inference, APA Board of Scientific Affairs. Statistical methods in psychology journals: guidelines and explanations. *Am Psychol.* 1999;54:594–604.
12. Hawkes N. *Early Scientific Instruments.* New York: Abbeville Press; 1981.
13. Munro BH, Page EB. *Statistical Methods for Health Care Research.* 2nd ed. Philadelphia: JB Lippincott; 1993.
14. Baumgardner KR. A review of key research design and statistical analysis issues. *Oral Surg Oral Med Oral Pathol.* 1997;84:550–556.
15. Skolnick BE. Ethical and institutional review board issues. *Adv Neurol.* 1998;76:253–262.
16. U.S. Department of Health and Human Services. Protection of human subjects. 45 CFR §46.
17. Flanagin A. Who wrote the Declaration of Helsinki? *JAMA.* 1997;277:926.
18. Declaration of Helsinki: Recommendations guiding physicians in biomedical research involving human subjects. *JAMA.* 1997;277:925–926.
19. Montgomery C, Lydon A, Lloyd K. Patients may not understand enough to give their informed consent [Letter, Comment]. *BMJ.* 1997;314:1482.
20. Hayes KW. Making tests with low reliability work for you. *Orthop Pract.* 1999;11:28–29,35.
21. Fischer EP. Art and science. *Nature.* 1997;390:330.
22. Cohen J. *Statistical Power Analysis for the Behavioral Sciences.* 2nd ed. Hillsdale, N.J.: Erlbaum; 1988.
23. Witte RS, Witte JS. *Statistics.* 5th ed. Fort Worth, Tex: Harcourt Brace College; 1997.
24. Welkowitz J, Ewen RB, Cohen J. *Introductory Statistics for the Behavioral Sciences.* 4th ed. Fort Worth, Tex: Harcourt Brace Jovanovich College; 1991.
25. Gehlbach SH. *Interpreting the Medical Literature.* 3rd ed. New York: McGraw-Hill; 1993.
26. Angell M, Kassirer JP. Clinical research: what should the public believe? [Editorial.] *N Engl J Med.* 1994;331:189–190.

27. Greenfield MLVH, Kuhn JE, Wojtys EM. A statistics primer. *Am J Sports Med.* 1996;24:393–395.

28. Hillway T. *Introduction to Research.* 2nd ed. Boston: Houghton Mifflin; 1964.

29. Watson GD, Crick FHC. Molecular structure of nucleic acids: a structure for deoxyribose nucleic acid. *Nature.* 1953;171:737.

30. Taylor A. The jargon in nursing journals. *Nurs Times.* 1998;94:47.

31. Armstrong SJ. Unintelligible management research and academic prestige. *Interfaces.* 1980;10:80–86.

32. Crichton M. Medical obfuscation: structure and function. *N Engl J Med.* 1975;293:1257–1259.

22

Where to Find It in a Report

It may help to know where to find parts of a research report (Figure 22-1), therefore, the report's section below has been numbered and highlighted with a marker as a guide. As an exercise, it may be useful to look at a highlighted area first, and then determine whether you can identify the portion of the report to which it belongs.

Prelims

1. Title
2. Authors
3. Affiliations
4. Abstract

Introduction

5. The general problem
6. The specific issue
7. The theoretical need for the study
8. The problem statement
9. The null hypothesis

Method

10. Subject selection and criteria*
11. Description of instruments
12. Validity and reliability of the instruments
13. Standardized procedures for collecting data
14. A photograph of the experimental setup
15. A description of the design
16. Choice of statistical analysis and α level

Results

17. Descriptive analysis of the three dependent variables
18. Tables containing descriptive analyses of the three dependent variables
19. Transformation of raw scores because of violated statistical assumptions (skewed distribution)
20. Inferential statistics and null hypothesis revisited
21. Supplementary analysis to explore other relationships not planned for at the beginning of the study
22. Limitations of supplementary findings

Discussion

23. Theory identified to make sense of the primary findings in study
24. Support from other studies and neuroanatomy
25. Lack of support from other studies possibly attributed to use of different methods
26. Support of supplementary findings from other studies

Conclusions

27. Primary findings
28. Need for future studies of the topic explored in the supplementary analysis

Acknowledgments

29. Funding source and support from individuals
30. Address for correspondences to author

References

31. References to credit the work of others

---

* Power analysis reported in dissertation: Batavia M. The effect of circumferential wrist pressure on reproduction accuracy of wrist placement in healthy young and elderly adults [dissertation]. New York: New York University; 1997.

Journal of Gerontology: MEDICAL SCIENCES
1999, Vol. 54A, No. 4, M177–M183

Copyright 1999 by The Gerontological Society of America

The Effects of Circumferential Wrist Pressure on Reproduction Accuracy of Wrist Placement in Healthy Young and Elderly Adults

Mitchell Batavia,[1] John G. Gianutsos,[2] Wen Ling,[1] and Arthur J. Nelson[3]

[1]Department of Physical Therapy, School of Education, New York University.
[2]Department of Rehabilitation Medicine, New York University Medical Center.
[3]Physical Therapy Program, College of Staten Island, City University of New York.

Background. The purpose of this study was to determine the effect of circumferential wrist pressure on reproduction accuracy of wrist placement in healthy young and elderly adults. A convenience sample of 20 young adults having a mean age of 22.9 years and 20 elderly adults with a mean age of 68.2 years participated in the study.

Method. Blindfolded subjects were asked to actively self-select a neutral wrist position (reference) and then, when signaled, to actively reproduce the previously selected position. Wrist joint reproduction accuracy was assessed under four pressure conditions: no contact, wrist contact, 10 mm Hg, and 20 mm Hg. A single axis dynamic wrist electrogoniometer measured three dependent variables: absolute, constant, and variable errors. Data were analyzed by means of multivariate analysis of variance (MANOVA) for repeated measures.

Results. No significant differences in reproduction accuracy under the four pressure conditions for young or elderly adults were found.

Conclusions. Healthy young and elderly adults may utilize existing intrinsic feedback and central control mechanisms to achieve accuracy during a reproduction task. Some subjects in both age groups who entered into the study with high error scores benefited from circumferential pressure by possibly relying on peripheral mechanisms. Further studies are needed to determine the effect of circumferential pressure on subjects with poor reproduction performance.

PHYSICAL rehabilitation specialists are interested in methods of enhancing motor performance in individuals whose functional abilities are limited. Previous studies using passive–active testing paradigms report improved joint position accuracy when circumferential pressure is applied around the knee joint (1–6) or ankle joint (7–9). Enhancing joint position sense is relevant in rehabilitation because of its importance in motor learning, balance, and injury prevention (1,4,5) and may be especially relevant to elderly persons reliant on joint position sense in the dark when they are prone to falls and resultant injuries.

Previous studies used passive–active paradigms that entailed having the subject actively match a joint position passively specified by the experimenter. Subjects tested under these conditions may be more reliant on afferent (sensory) feedback for accurate limb placement. Feuerbach and colleagues (7) postulated that pressure application at the ankle improves joint position sense by increasing afferent (sensory) feedback from cutaneous receptors.

Passive–active paradigms place insufficient emphasis on the fact that position sense is influenced by both peripheral and central (motor outflow) contributions (10). In humans, muscle spindle activity, critical to proprioception, does not operate independently of its gamma efferents (11). Hence, muscle spindles are dynamically active during motion. Moreover, cutaneous input is inhibited by voluntary movement (12). Furthermore, passive–active paradigms do not simulate real-life challenges and, therefore, are difficult to generalize to activities of daily living (13). Shortcomings of previous studies include a lack of controlled pressure application around the joint (1–9) and have unknown instrumental validity (1,4,5,6,8).

A review of the literature has not revealed studies investigating the effect of circumferential pressure on active–active reproduction accuracy of limb position. Active–active paradigms require the subject to actively match a limb position to a target actively selected by the subject (preselection). Subjects tested with such a reproduction task may rely primarily on efferent (motor) signals derived from motor programs originating from the central nervous system and less so on afferent (sensory) feedback accompanying accurate limb placement (13). Although an age-related decline in position sense measured at a single joint has been demonstrated using passive–active matching paradigms (1,5,14–18), age may not be a factor in accuracy of joint placement under active–active conditions.

The purpose of this study was to determine if age or circumferential pressure affects accuracy of a motor task under active–active conditions. This study addressed the theoretical basis of sensory input on movement accuracy during a voluntary movement to determine if enhanced sources of afferent feedback facilitate motor control during active movement. No differences in reproduction accuracy between young and elderly adults or under the four pressure conditions for either age group were expected.

METHOD

Subjects.—A convenience sample of 20 healthy young and 20 healthy elderly adult volunteers between the ages of 18–30 and 60–75 years, respectively, was recruited through local advertisements and flyers in the New York City metropolitan area.

M177

Figure 22-1. Report of a peer-reviewed quasiexperimental study. *(From Batavia M, Gianutsos JG, Ling W, Nelson AJ. The effects of circumferential wrist pressure on reproduction accuracy of wrist placement in healthy young and elderly adults. J Gerontol Med Sci. 1999;54A:M177–M183. Reprinted with permission from the Journal of Gerontology.)*

⑩ Ten men and 10 women served as subjects in each age group. With the exception of one young adult, all were right-hand dominant. Exclusion criteria included the presence of neurological disease, vascular disease, or musculoskeletal problems in the dominant upper extremity. This study was approved by the New York University Medical Center's Institutional Review Board. Informed consent was obtained from all subjects, who were paid twenty dollars for participating.

Instrumentation.—A single axis dynamic wrist electrogoniometer was utilized to measure movement reproduction accuracy in the sagittal plane. This type of device is reported to be accurate, reliable, and useful in controlled laboratory investigations involving a single joint (19) and in functional wrist movement studies (20). The electrogoniometer used in this study did not provide contact cues over the wrist area and provided less than 1 mm Hg of pressure over the forearm across all conditions.

The electrogoniometer, constructed by bioengineers at NYU Medical Center, weighed 7 ounces and consisted of parallelogram-configured metal rods linked to a potentiometer mounted on a dorsal and forearm piece. Movements of the electrogoniometer falling within a 165-degree range resulted in a voltage output from the potentiometer, which was converted to a joint angle measurement (0.0225 volts = 1.0 degree) by means ⑪ of a position sense software.

An aneroid sphygmomanometer, which delivered and measured circumferential wrist pressure, consisted of a newborn inflation bag and cuff of 1.5-inch width (Tycos Instruments, Model 5082–07, Arden, NC), hollow rubber tubing, a plastic T fitting, an inflation bulb, an aneroid pressure gauge, and a Velcro strap. The inflation bulb filled the inflation bag with air at pressures indicated by the gauge. The aneroid sphygmomanometer detects pressures ranging from 0 to 300 mm Hg in 2 mm Hg intervals. Pressures ranging from 0 to 20 mm Hg were utilized in this study.

Concurrent validity of the electrogoniometer was determined by comparing its voltage output with values obtained from a clinical goniometer attached to the hand and forearm piece of the electrogoniometer. Concurrent validity, ICC $(2,1) = .99$, $p < .001$, and test–retest reliability, ICC $(2,1) = .99$, $p < .001$, data of the electrogoniometer were good, as determined by intraclass correlation coefficients. The standard error of measurement (*SEM*) of the electrogoniometer on repeated measures for eight ⑫ angles (within the measurement range of the study) was small, ranging from 0.023 to 0.052 with a median *SEM* of 0.026. The electrogoniometer had an absolute error of 0.4 degrees.

Concurrent validity of the aneroid sphygmomanometer was determined by attaching and comparing measurements of the aneroid sphygmomanometer with a mercurial sphygmomanometer. Concurrent validity and test–retest reliability of the pressure gauge were good, ICC $(2,1) = .99$, $p < .001$, and ICC $(2,1) = 1.0$, $p < .001$, respectively. Concurrent validity of the electrogoniometer and aneroid sphygmomanometer was reconfirmed at the completion of the study.

Procedures.—To ensure consistency of procedures, a checklist was followed. Subjects were randomly assigned to one of four ⑬ possible pressure sequences. Then they completed a demographic and health questionnaire, an Orientation-Memory-Concentration test [OMCT; (21)], a physical activity question-

naire [PAQ; (22)], and a physical screening of the dominant upper extremity. The physical screening, which was performed by a licensed physical therapist, included tests for carpal tunnel syndrome (Phalen's test, Tinel's test, pinch test), test for light touch, position sense, manual muscle test, range of motion, two-point discrimination, and diminished light touch using monofilaments.

The experimental setup is shown in Figure 1. Subjects sat in a chair with their dominant forearm undraped and supported on a table. The upper extremity position was standardized and maintained for all conditions with the elbow in 165 degrees of extension, the forearm in pronation and horizontally stabilized on a foam support. The wrist, which was positioned beyond the front edge of the support, was free to flex and extend.

The electrogoniometer was secured across the subject's palm and forearm with Velcro straps; it was not in contact with the wrist joint, and it remained on the subject's upper extremity throughout the entire experiment. The sphygmomanometer cuff was centered and secured over the distal volar wrist crease at the wrist. Consistent positioning of both instruments was confirmed during and between pressure conditions using skin markings.

While blindfolded, subjects were familiarized with the testing procedure through 10 practice trials. Each trial consisted of a subject-selected reference and reproduction response. Each subject was given standardized verbal instructions. For the reference measurement, the subject was instructed to begin from a position of wrist flexion and to extend the wrist within a one-second period to a self-selected middle (neutral) position set within a 16-degree range determined through software. Next, the subject was instructed to reproduce the reference wrist joint position movement as accurately as possible by repeating the procedure without a rest period. A 15-second rest period was instituted between trials to avoid fatigue.

Following the practice trials, the subject completed 10 trials for each of the four pressure conditions, separated by a one-minute rest period, utilizing the procedures described during the practice trial. Between trials and conditions, subjects returned their wrists to a relaxed, flexed angle with fingers relaxed and open. Wrist position and relaxation were confirmed with electrogoniometer output and palpation, respectively. For the no-wrist-contact condition, a sphygmomanometer cuff was not used. For the contact condition, the cuff contacted the sub-

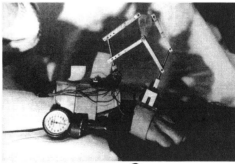

Figure 1. The experimental setup.

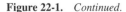

Figure 22-1.   *Continued.*

ject's skin with the gauge needle indicator output at 0.00 mm Hg. For the mild pressure condition, the cuff was inflated to 10 mm Hg while the wrist was actively maintained in a neutral position. For the moderate pressure condition, the cuff was secured around the subject's wrist as previously indicated with the bag inflated to 20 mm Hg. Pressure during the last two conditions was maintained by use of a hemostat.

Design.—A 2 × 4 repeated measures design with a between-groups factor of age and a within factor of pressure was utilized. A balanced 4 × 4 Latin square served to counterbalance the sequence of pressure conditions for each age group (23).

Data analysis.—For each trial, peak wrist joint extension was recorded for both reference and reproduction measurements. An error score, in degrees, was derived by subtracting the reference measurement from the reproduction measurement. The error scores from the 10 trials were then averaged to calculate a subject's absolute error (AE), constant error (CE), and variable error (VE) for each condition using the unsigned differences, signed differences, and the standard deviation of the signed differences, respectively (24). Consonant with similar studies to effect comparisons, absolute, constant, and variable errors were calculated. These measurements provide information regarding the accuracy, bias, and consistency of achieving a target, respectively.

Because elderly adults have been reported to undershoot targets when tested during passive–active paradigms, constant errors were analyzed (15,16).

Data were analyzed utilizing a multivariate analysis of variance (MANOVA) with an alpha level set at .05 using the Statistical Program for the Social Sciences (SPSS), Advanced Windows version 6.1.2 (SPSS Inc., Chicago, IL).

RESULTS

Table 1 shows group demographics and performance on the PAQ and the OMCT. Young and elderly adults performed similarly on the PAQ, implying that the two groups had similar physical activity levels. OMCT scores, although significantly different with t tests for independent groups, $t = 2.02$, $p = .05$, indicated no memory deficit in either group. No differences between age groups were found for two-point discrimination at the wrist with t tests for independent groups, $t = 0.08$, $p = .93$.

Table 2 contains raw absolute error scores of the young and elderly adults for the four pressure conditions. Mean absolute error scores for elderly adults were smaller than those of young adult scores under all pressure conditions. Errors were greatest for both groups during the no-contact condition and smallest for both groups under moderate pressure conditions.

Raw constant error scores of the young and elderly adults for the four pressure conditions are presented in Table 3. In con-

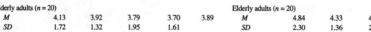

Table 1. Group Demographics

Variable	Young ($n = 20$)	Elderly ($n = 20$)	Total ($N = 40$)	t test	p value
Age					
M	22.90	68.20	45.55	–34.77	.000
SD	3.31	4.79	23.29		
PAQ*					
M	10.32	9.54	9.93	0.42	.67
SD	6.13	5.49	5.76		
OMCT†					
M	1.25	2.45	1.85	–2.02	.05
SD	1.80	1.96	1.96		

*Physical Activities Questionnaire.
†Orientation Memory Concentration Test.

Table 3. Summary of Means and Standard Deviations of Raw Constant Errors (degrees) for Young and Elderly Adults During Four Pressure Conditions

	1 No Contact	2 Contact	3 Mild Pressure	4 Moderate Pressure	Mean
Young adults ($n = 20$)					
M	0.80	0.81	0.17	0.74	0.63
SD	3.29	2.49	3.07	2.08	
Elderly adults ($n = 20$)					
M	0.62	1.96	1.00	1.00	1.14
SD	2.23	2.32	2.35	2.45	
Total ($N = 40$)					
M	0.71	1.39	0.58	0.87	0.89

Table 2. Summary of Means and Standard Deviations of Raw Absolute Errors (degrees) for Young and Elderly Adults During Four Pressure Conditions

	1 No Contact	2 Contact	3 Mild Pressure	4 Moderate Pressure	Mean
Young adults ($n = 20$)					
M	4.68	4.23	4.39	4.12	4.35
SD	1.76	1.20	1.45	1.84	
Elderly adults ($n = 20$)					
M	4.13	3.92	3.79	3.70	3.89
SD	1.72	1.32	1.95	1.61	
Total ($N = 40$)					
M	4.40	4.07	4.09	3.91	4.12

Table 4. Summary of Means and Standard Deviations of Raw Variable Errors (degrees) for Young and Elderly Adults During Four Pressure Conditions

	1 No Contact	2 Contact	3 Mild Pressure	4 Moderate Pressure	Mean
Young adults ($n = 20$)					
M	5.27	4.75	4.66	4.84	4.88
SD	1.94	1.47	1.59	2.74	
Elderly adults ($n = 20$)					
M	4.84	4.33	4.29	4.06	4.38
SD	2.30	1.36	2.23	1.56	
Total ($N = 40$)					
M	5.05	4.54	4.48	4.45	4.63

Figure 22-1. *Continued.*

trast to absolute error patterns, mean constant error scores for elderly adults were greater than those of young adults for all pressure conditions except for the no-contact condition.

Raw variable error scores of the young and elderly adults for the four pressure conditions are shown in Table 4. For the elderly adult group, variable error patterns were similar to the absolute error trend with progressively smaller errors occurring with increasing pressure.

Data transformations.—Raw variable errors were positively skewed for all pressure conditions and responded well to log 10 transformations. Consequently, log 10 transformed variable error scores were used in the analyses. In contrast, raw absolute and constant error scores were analyzed in their original untransformed states.

Inferential statistics.—A MANOVA was used because the dependent variables were correlated (23) and the data showed appropriate homogeneity (25). The results of the MANOVA indicate that the two groups behaved similarly. No significant differences were obtained regarding reproduction accuracy of wrist placement during the four pressure conditions in healthy young adults, in healthy elderly adults, or between healthy young and elderly adults under the four conditions. Between-subjects main effects of age group were not significant [$F(3,36) = 0.96$, $p = .42$]. Within-subjects main effect of pressure was not significant [$F(9,30) = 0.83$, $p = .59$]. The interaction effect of Age $\times$ Pressure was not significant [$F(9,30)$, $p = .56$]. Furthermore, a repeated measures ANOVA revealed no statistically significant differences for sequence [$F(3,114) = .45$, $p = .72$], implying that a practice effect did not occur. Finally, no relationship was found between the variability in a subject's choice of target location and absolute error scores in the 40 subjects, suggesting that accuracy was not related to the subject's consistency in choosing a reference target.

Supplementary analyses.—In a previous study, Perlau and colleagues (4) noted a 66% improvement in position sense at the knee of healthy adults (ages 22–40) following pressure application if the subject had a pre-bandage error score of 5 degrees or more. A trend was also noted in this study, in that sub-jects who entered into the study with higher absolute error scores (no-contact condition) tended to demonstrate greater reduction in errors with mild pressure. This suggests that these individuals benefited most from pressure application (Figure 2).

Subjects were therefore regrouped, regardless of age, into a low error group ($n = 26$) if they scored below 5 degrees of error during the baseline (no-contact) condition or into a high error group ($n = 14$) if they scored at or above 5 degrees of error during the baseline (no-contact) condition (4). Of the 14 subjects in the high error group, 8 were young adults and 6 were elderly adults. There was no significant relationship between age and square root transformed absolute error scores in the high error group, $r = .01$, $p = .97$ or the low error group, $r = -.17$, $p = .38$.

Means for low and high group raw absolute errors during the four pressure conditions are plotted in Figure 3 and reveal a small increase in errors for the low error group and a large decrease in errors for the high error group under the mild pressure condition. Absolute errors were square root transformed because of significant positively skewed distributions.

Although significant, MANOVA was not conducted because the multivariate Boxs M test for homogeneity was not satisfied (25). Rather, to explore the effect of circumferential pressure on high and low error groups, a two-way repeated measures ANOVA with one between (error group) one within (pressure) was conducted.

Unweighted square root absolute error means (unique sums of square) were used in the analysis because of unequal sample size. Homogeneity of variance tests was not significant for the two-way ANOVA. A nonsignificant Mauchly sphericity test indicated that the assumption of compound symmetry was satisfied. Error Group $\times$ Pressure interactions were significant $F(3,114) = 5.32$, $p = .002$. Simple main effects were significant for the high error group ($n = 14$), $F(3,114) = 5.88$, $p < .01$, but not for the low error group ($n = 26$), $F(3,114) = 0.59$, $p > .05$.

Post hoc Tukey tests were significant only for the high error group between the no-contact and mild pressure and the no-contact and moderate pressure conditions. The two error groups were significantly different under the no-contact condition [$F(1,38) = 98.52$, $p < .001$] and wrist contact condition [$F(1,38) = 24.14$, $p < .001$]. The two error groups were not significantly different under the mild pressure condition [$F(1,38) = 1.6$, $p = .21$] or using a Mann-Whitney comparison, under the moderate

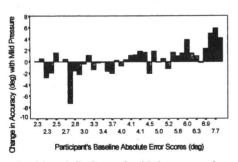

Figure 2. Bar graph of baseline untransformed absolute error scores under no contact conditions and change in absolute error scores during mild circumferential pressure conditions ($N = 40$).

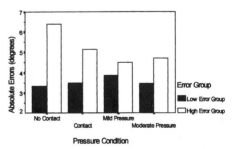

Figure 3. Absolute error of low and high error groups during four pressure conditions.

Figure 22-1. *Continued.*

pressure condition, suggesting that performance of the high error group improved relative to that of the low error group with mild and moderate circumferential pressure. It should be noted that for the high error group, either a practice effect or a regression to the mean is possible.

Finally, *t* tests yielded no significant differences between the high and low error groups on the PAQ, two-point discrimination, wrist joint range of motion, or OMCT scores.

DISCUSSION

Central mechanisms and movement reproduction.—This study showed that circumferential wrist pressure did not universally affect reproduction accuracy of wrist placement in healthy young or elderly adults during an active–active paradigm. As detailed in Tables 2 through 4, differences between elderly and young adults' errors were small and not statistically significant. An active–active testing paradigm was used, and for some, but not all subjects, information from motor outputs and existing intrinsic feedback was sufficient to enhance accuracy during the task. Note that one source of variance may be related to the fact that an electrogoniometer was used in this study. Camera-based motion analysis was not used in the present study because unwanted contact cues emanating from the reflective markers, which are applied directly over the joint of interest, would confound the effects of pressure application. In addition, Klein and DeHaven (26) report that motion analysis systems inherently increase measurement error as a neutral position (i.e., 180 degrees) is approached (a joint position well within the range used in this study).

The theories of Kelso and Wallace (13) hold that active–active testing paradigms rely predominantly on central motor control mechanisms through corollary-discharge signals present during active target selection.

In this study, active testing may have enabled subjects to process incoming information about target location efficiently during both phases of the task. Stelmach and Sirica (17) also maintain that corollary discharge has a preselection effect for target location, whereby motor signals prepare sensory mechanisms for the sensory consequences of movement.

Neuroanatomic pathways that support the corollary discharge hypothesis include ascending flexor reflex afferent (FRA) paths and extensive interconnections between the motor cortex and anterior lobe of the cerebellum (27). In addition, descending control of muscle spindles provides a central (efferent) control mechanism for maintaining sensitivity of muscle spindles length and can ensure continued supply of information about muscle length to higher centers (28).

The present findings are consonant with those of upper extremity movement reproduction studies in humans in which healthy subjects demonstrated significantly lower errors in the reproduction task only during an active condition (29–30). Our findings are also consistent with multi-joint upper extremity displacement studies in which intrinsic feedback, reportedly diminished in the elderly subjects (31), did not affect accuracy in the elderly adults as compared to the accuracy of young adults under active testing conditions (17,18). According to Stelmach and Sirica (17), central control mechanisms operating during preselected movements can compensate for diminished proprioception in elderly adults by enhancing the encoding of information about the sensory consequences of movement. Previous

studies that have found age-related position sense differences have tested subjects under passive conditions, where central control mechanisms may not be invoked. In contrast, no age-related differences in the reproduction task were found in the present study, because the active–active paradigm allows access to utilization of central control mechanisms.

Age seems to be a factor in determining accuracy of movement reproduction under passive conditions. Both Meeuwsen and colleagues (16) and Kaplan and colleagues (15) noted that elderly adults tend to undershoot target position during passive testing. These researchers speculate that the elderly adults attempt to monitor their movements to a greater extent than young adults by relying on sensory feedback (15).

Although comparison of elderly adults' performance during passive movement was not examined in the present study, one could speculate that elderly people may operate under different modes of control during active testing versus passive testing. Under passive testing conditions, the elders may be monitoring their performance, albeit with diminished peripheral feedback, resulting in a more cautious performance and greater underestimation of joint targets as compared with a younger adult group. However, under active testing procedures used in the present study, elderly adults actually overshot their targets more so than young adults. The healthy elderly group may have been relying on motor programs requiring less monitoring during performance, thereby resulting in less cautious performance than is more characteristic of the young adult group.

The findings in the present study contradict those in previous research found under passive testing conditions comparing position sense accuracy of young and elderly adults (1,5,14,16). Age-related neurological and morphological changes found in elderly adults (31,32) have been postulated as the cause of diminished proprioceptive performances in elders. Proprioceptive performance in the elderly group, however, was commonly tested passively in previous studies (4), thereby negating the important contribution of central control mechanisms (such as corollary discharge) to proprioception during voluntary movement. Few functional activities in life are analogous to passive position sense tests (10,13). Testing under active conditions may better simulate conditions that approximate real life, such as reaching, transferring, or walking in dark surroundings. From this viewpoint, it is more reasonable to test proprioception in elderly adults using an active–active paradigm in order to assess the contribution of central control mechanisms to enhance functional performance.

Peripheral mechanisms and movement reproduction.—Supplementary analysis in this study was prompted by previously reported findings that subjects with poorer position sense may derive greater benefit from circumferential pressure than those with good position sense. Error is one of a number of ways that subjects could have been assigned to groups. The findings in this study suggest that the subject's entering performance may determine whether sensory feedback sources augment movement accuracy during voluntary movement. Regardless of age, joint reproduction accuracy was enhanced through sensory feedback derived from circumferential pressure in subjects entering with high error scores, and failed to be enhanced in their low error entering performance counterparts.

As Figure 3 illustrates, additional sensory input reduced absolute errors (1.90 degrees) in the high error group, but increased

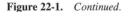

Figure 22-1. *Continued.*

them slightly (0.54 degrees) in the low error group. Subjects having higher entering error scores may have engaged (i.e., been more actively involved) in the task only when additional augmented feedback in the form of circumferential pressure was imposed.

The findings in the supplementary analyses of this study are consistent with the results of Perlau and colleagues (4) in which a 66% improvement in position sense resulted following elastic bandage application in a poor position sense group, whereas no measurable changes were found in the good position sense group. Interestingly, individuals in the present study who entered with low error scores did not tend to benefit, and in some cases even deteriorated during pressure application (Figure 2). This trend substantiates Perlau and coworkers' (4) suggestion that enhanced afferent stimulation may serve to confuse individuals who have inherently good position sense. Possible detrimental effects of sensory feedback have been demonstrated with visual (13), auditory (31,) and cutaneous inputs as well (12).

Other studies have shown the efficacy of circumferential pressure on position sense in patients with osteoarthritis or total knee replacements who tested poorly on position sense (1,5). In contrast, following elastic bandage application, position sense was not improved in subjects with good position sense.

The notion of improved accuracy with augmented sensory feedback in high error groups is not without merit when one considers the importance of proprioceptive inputs, derived from cutaneous, joint, and muscle spindle receptors to joint position sense (33), or that cutaneous afferents are the defining input for proprioception (34). Cutaneous mechanoreceptors have both a facilitative (35) and specific role (36) in position sense. Rapidly adapting receptors may respond to dynamic stimuli such as the movement of a bandage over the skin (2,4). Slowly adapting receptors, such as Ruffini cutaneous receptors, may provide both static and dynamic proprioceptive input in response to pressure (4).

Evarts (37) studied monkeys and found that kinesthetic inputs involve short latency responses to and from cerebral cortex of the order of 35 msec. This suggests that there is sufficient time for kinesthetic inputs to influence motor output during voluntary movements. It is therefore entirely possible that during the present study, there was adequate time for peripheral mechanisms to influence movement reproduction.

Conclusions.—Healthy young and elderly adults do not differ in their ability to actively reproduce a wrist movement and may utilize existing intrinsic feedback and central control mechanisms to achieve accuracy during a reproduction task. Circumferential pressure did not enhance accuracy in either age group.

Some subjects in both age groups who entered into the study with high error scores may have benefited from circumferential pressure, possibly by relying on peripheral mechanisms. However, because the present study was not designed to examine the effects of circumferential pressure on reproduction accuracy in high and low error groups, further studies, using active–active paradigms in a planned comparison, are needed. In addition, studies that examine the effect of circumferential pressure on reproduction accuracy in individuals with central nervous system disorders are warranted.

ACKNOWLEDGMENTS

This work was funded in part by a grant from the U.S. Department of Education, National Institute of Disability and Rehabilitation Research for physical therapy clinical research. It was accepted as an abstract and platform presentation at the APTA Physical Therapy 1998 Scientific Meeting and Exposition, Orlando, FL.

We gratefully acknowledge Dr. Sharon L. Weinberg for her feedback on statistical analyses; Carl Mason and Aaron Beattie for their technical support of instrumentation and computer programs; Linda Medford for her assistance in the fabrication of material for the electrogoniometer; and Christine K. Wade for her English translation of a German journal article.

This study was completed in partial fulfillment of the requirements for Dr. Batavia's Doctor of Philosophy degree in the School of Education, New York University.

Address correspondence to Dr. Mitchell Batavia, Department of Physical Therapy, New York University, 380 Second Avenue, 4th floor, New York, NY 10010. E-mail: mitchell.batavia@nyu.edu

REFERENCES

1. Barrett DS, Cobb A, Bentley G. Joint proprioception in normal, osteoarthritic and replaced knees. *J Bone Joint Surg.* 1991;73B:53–56.
2. Jerosch J, Prymka M. Propriozeptive fähigkeiten des gesunden kniegelenks: Beeinflussung durch eine elastische bandage [in German]. *Sportverletzung. Sportschaden.* 1995;9:72–76.
3. McNair PJ, Stanley SN, Strauss GR. Knee bracing: effects on proprioception. *Arch Phys Med Rehabil.* 1996;77:287–289.
4. Perlau R, Frank C, Flick G. The effect of elastic bandages on human knee proprioception in the uninjured population. *Am J Sports Med.* 1995;23: 251–255.
5. Sell S, Zacher J, Lack S. Propriozeptionsstörung am arthrotischen kniegelenk [in German]. *Zeitschrift für Rheumatologie.* 1993;52:150–155.
6. Jerosch J, Prymka M, Castro WHM. Proprioception of knee joints with a lesion of the medial mensicus. *Acta Orthopaedica Belgica.* 1996;62:41–45.
7. Feuerbach JW, Grabiner MD, Koh TJ, Weiker GG. Effect of an ankle orthosis and ankle ligament anesthesia on ankle joint proprioception. *Am J Sports Med.* 1994; 22, 223–229.
8. Jerosch J, Hoffstetter I, Bork H, Bischof M. The influence of orthoses on the proprioception of the ankle. *Knee Surgery, Sports Traumatology, Arthroscopy.* 1995;3:39–46.
9. Zablonski GL. *The Effect of Ankle Bracing and Taping on Proprioception.* Buffalo, NY: D'Youville College; 1994. Master's thesis.
10. Matthews PBC. Proprioceptors and their contribution to somatosensory mapping: complex messages require complex processing. *Can J Physiol Pharmacol.* 1988;66:430–438.
11. Brooks VB. *The Neural Basis of Motor Control.* New York: Oxford University Press; 1986.
12. Coquery J–M. Role of active movement in control of afferent input from skin in cat and man. In: Gordon G, ed. *Active Touch.* Elmsford, NY: Pergamon; 1978:161–169.
13. Kelso JAS, Wallace SA. Conscious mechanisms in movement. In: Stelmach GE, ed. *Information Processing in Motor Control and Learning.* New York: Academic Press, 1978: 79–116.
14. Skinner HB, Barrack RL, Cook SD. Age related decline in proprioception. *Clin Orthopaed Related Res.* 1984;184:208–211.
15. Kaplan FS, Nixon JE, Reitz M, Rindfleish L, Tucker J. Age related changes in proprioception and sensation of joint position. *Acta Orthop Scand.* 1985;56:72–74.
16. Meeuwsen HJ, Sawicki TM, Stelmach GE. Improved foot position sense as a result of repetition in older adults. *J Gerontol Psych Sci.* 1993;48: P137–P141.
17. Stelmach GE, Sirica A. Aging and proprioception. *Age.* 1986;9:99–103.
18. Dick MB, Kean M–L, Sands D. The preselection effect on the recall facilitation of motor movements in Alzheimer's-type dementia. *J Gerontol Psych Sci.* 1988;43:P127–P135.
19. Ladin Z. Three-dimensional instrumentation. In: Allard P, Stokes IAF, Blanchi J-P, eds. *Three-Dimensional Analysis of Human Movement.* Champaign, IL: Human Kinetics; 1995.
20. Ryu J, Palmer AK, Cooney WP. Wrist joint motion. In: An K-N, Berger RA, Cooney WP, eds. *Biomechanics of the Wrist Joint.* New York: Springer-Verlag; 1991:37–60.
21. Katzman R, Brown T, Fuld P, Peck A, Schechter R, Schimmel H. Validation of a short Orientation-Memory-Concentration Test of cognitive impairment. *Am J Psychiatry.* 1983;140:734–739.
22. Voorrips LE, Ravelli ACJ, Dongelmans PCA, Deurenberg P, Staveren WAV. A physical activity questionnaire for the elderly. *Med Sci Sports Exerc.* 1990;23:974–979.

Figure 22-1.   *Continued.*

23. Portney LG, Watkins MP. *Foundations of Clinical Research: Applications to Practice.* Norwalk, CT: Appleton & Lange; 1993.

24. Magill RA. *Motor Learning: Concepts and Applications.* 4th ed. Madison, WI: WCB Brown & Benchmark; 1993.

25. Tebacknick BG, Fidell LS. *Using Multivariate Statistics.* 2nd ed. Northridge, NY: Harper & Row; 1989.

26. Klein JP, Dehaven JJ. Accuracy of three-dimensional linear and angular estimates obtained with the Ariel Performance Analysis System. *Arch Phys Med Rehabil.* 1995;76:183–189.

27. Evarts EV. Feedback and corollary discharge: a merging of the concepts. *Neurosci Res Prog Bull.* 1971;9:89–112.

28. Phillips CG. Motor apparatus of the baboon's hand. *Proc R Soc Lond.* 1968;173:141–174.

29. Kelso JAS. Planning and efferent components in the coding of movement. *J Motor Behav.* 1977;1:33–47.

30. Stelmach GE, Kelso JAS, Wallace SA. Preselection in short-term motor memory. *J Exp Psychol: Hum Learning Mem.* 1975;1:745–755.

31. Levin HS, Benton AL. Age effects in proprioceptive feedback performance. *Gerontologia Clinica.* 1973;15:161–169.

32. Sabin TD, Venna N. Peripheral nerve disorders in the elderly. In: Albert, ML, ed. *Clinical Neurology of Aging.* New York: Oxford University Press; 1984:425–442.

33. Gandevia SC, Hall LA, McCloskey, DI, Potter, E. K. Proprioceptive sensation at the terminal joint of the middle finger. *J Physiol.* 1983;335:507–517.

34. Moberg E. The role of cutaneous afferents in position sense, kinaesthesia, and motor function of the hand. *Brain.* 1983;106:1–19.

35. Gandevia SC, McCloskey DI. Joint sense, muscle sense, and their combination as position sense, measured at the distal interphalangeal joint of the middle finger. *J Physiol.* 1976;260:387–407.

36. Edin BB. Quantitative analysis of static strain sensitivity in human mechanoreceptors from hairy skin. *J Neurophysiol.* 1992;67:1105–1113.

37. Evarts EV. Sensorimotor cortex activity associated with movements triggered by visual as compared to somesthetic inputs. In: Schmitt FO, Worden FG, eds. *The Neurosciences: Third Study Program.* Cambridge, MA: MIT Press; 1974: 327–337.

Received August 22, 1997
Accepted May 28, 1998

Figure 22-1.   *Continued.*

Part V

Clinicians and Graduate Students

Chapters 23 through 25 discuss some of the separate concerns and interests of clinicians and graduate student researchers. The hope is that the gap between clinicians and researchers will narrow. Clinicians need to think more scientifically—that is, not to be persuaded by sellers of snake oil, such as some continuing education courses—and researchers need to ask more clinically relevant research questions.

23

Just for Clinicians

The purpose of this chapter is to assist clinicians who may want to become more involved in research activities but do not know where to begin. Although the material is geared to clinicians, graduate students may also benefit from this material. The following practical steps are discussed:

1. Starting a journal club
2. Establishing reliability in the clinic
3. Writing a case report
4. Sharing knowledge

STARTING A JOURNAL CLUB

The purpose of a journal club is to keep everyone in the clinic up to date with the knowledge of practice. Information from 5 to 10 years ago may no longer be valid. The goal is to review articles relevant to practice. Those working in a hand clinic will most likely review hand journals. Clinicians working in pediatrics may review journals on developmental disability.

How to run a journal club depends on the goals of the members, such as keeping current, improving critical appraisal of research, or enhancing patient care. One way is to have everyone review several current journal reports with a common theme one month before the meeting. Then each week one member can present one of the articles, and the others can critique it for strengths and weakness, overall believability, and relevance to the clinic. During the critique, the other assigned articles, including a classic publication in that area, can be brought up and woven into the fabric of the discussion so that the knowledge base can be assessed both from a current and historic perspective (J. Gianutsos, oral communication, May 2000). The main article should be evaluated for believability and clinical importance to patient care.

IMPROVING SUCCESS IN A JOURNAL CLUB

The following factors can enhance the success of a journal club.[1]

- Mandatory attendance
- Formal instruction by respected faculty members, as in biostatistics
- Refreshments
- A skilled moderator
- Reading guides or a checklist
- Use of principles of adult education, such as relating topics to patient care, active learning, and eclectic teaching formats
- Attendance by faculty members
- Perception that the program director acknowledges the educational importance of the club

CHECKLIST FOR JOURNAL CRITIQUE

The following checklist, derived from Chapter 21, can serve as a guide for journal club members.

Prelims

_____ Does the title broadcast the true nature of the study?

_____ Are the authors authorities on the research topic?

_____ Do the authors have a known bias, pet theory, or school of thought they are defending?

_____ Does the abstract summarize only findings contained within the study? (You may need to read the study and then reread the abstract.)

Introduction

_____ Is there adequate coverage to allow readers to appreciate the full scope of the problem?

_____ Are important journal citations omitted from the review, leading to a biased review?

_____ Is the clinical question important enough to escape the "so what?" reaction from readers?

_____ Are expected relationships between variables clearly stated before data collection was begun?

_____ If a description or association was sought, was an appropriate nonexperimental design used?

_____ If a cause-and-effect relationship was sought, was an appropriate experimental design used?

_____ Does the statistical analysis conducted match the type of data collected and design used?

_____ Was an α level set before data collection was begun?

Methods

_____ What population is identified in the study? Is this population important to your research or relevant to your clinical practice?

_____ Did sampling procedures enable recruitment of a representative sample of the population so that reasonable generalizations to that population can be made? (A convenience sample may limit such generalizations).

_____ Was the sample so large that _anyone_ would find a statistically significant result?

_____ Was the sample so small that _no one_ would find a statistically significant result?

_____ Was power analysis conducted to determine the sample size sufficient to find a statistically significant and important result if one exists?

_____ Was the setting controlled enough to ensure internal validity if a cause-and-effect relationship was being sought so that all factors except the one under study were controlled?

_____ Was the setting relevant enough to your practice to ensure some external validity?

_____ Are the validity and reliability of all measuring instruments reported as they relate to the population under study?

_____ Are the treatment procedures relevant to your research interests or clinical practice?

_____ Are procedures standardized to help enhance the internal validity of the experiment?

_____ Are procedures clear enough to allow replication?

Results

_____ Were statistical assumptions checked and satisfied (e.g., normal distribution of dependent variables) before hypothesis testing?

_____ Do the results seem plausible from an examination of the means, standard deviations, and graphs of the distributions?

_____ Are the results statistically significant, indicating that findings are reliable and probably not due to chance?

_____ Is the magnitude of change (effect size) impressive in terms of your research interests or clinical practice?

Discussion

_____ Do the authors attempt to fit the finding into the framework of previous findings?

_____ Do the authors make sense of the data and interpret them in terms of theory?

_____ Do the authors state any limitations or weaknesses of the study (all studies have some) or was it "a perfect study"?

_____ Do the authors confine their concluding remarks to the primary findings of the study, or do they only celebrate an unrelated finding that has no bearing on the original intent of the research?

Miscellaneous

_____ Are references dated, inaccurate, or not from primary sources, thus casting a shadow on the trustworthiness of these sources?

_____ Is the tone of the report an appeal to emotions rather than a presentation of evidence, suggesting that there is no objective basis for the conclusions?

_____ Is the report unintelligible or difficult to read, suggesting the authors may be trying to hide from or sidestep the facts?

_____ Do the funding sources for the study, such as drug companies, suggest a conflict of interest or potential bias in the study?

Draw your own conclusions about the credibility of the study and its importance to your practice.

ESTABLISHING RELIABILITY IN THE CLINIC

This section describes how to establish both intrarater and interrater reliability. Reliability is useful as an aid to clinical decision making, documenting patient care, or reporting a case. Conducting a reliability study is an excellent introduction to the research process. Instructions for conducting an analysis using a Pearson correlation and an intraclass correlation coefficient (ICC) will follow.

WHY ESTABLISH RELIABILITY IN THE CLINIC?

To determine whether patients truly improve over time, clinicians need to take consistent measurements. For example, if a patient's joint mobility measures 10 degrees greater at discharge than it was at admission, how can the clinician be certain the improvement is not caused by measurement error? Although reliability is emphasized in research education, it is not emphasized in clinical education. It is questionable whether most clinicians know how reliable or unreliable they are at assessing their patients. Because they can help determine whether a patient's condition improves or worsens over time, reliable measurements are an aid to clinical decision making.

Important: For the exercises in this chapter you will use existing patient information that you have collected as part of your normal weekly practice and documentation. Consult the institutional review board of your facility to determine whether you need approval for such research activities involving human subjects (see Chapter 21). I have used fictitious data.

ESTABLISHING INTRARATER RELIABILITY

It makes sense to establish intrarater reliability in your clinic if the same therapist takes all the measurements at initial and discharge evaluations. That way, the therapist will be confident that his or her measurements are recorded in a consistent manner from week to week. If a clinician wants to write a case report, establishing the reliability of the measuring tools in the report can strengthen the believability of the observations.

Objective

The objective is to determine how consistently you take measures on your patients. In the example, you want to find out whether you can consistently measure shoulder abduction with a goniometer for 10 patients with "frozen shoulders" on two separate occasions. Do measurements vary up or down in rank together? In reality, you can measure any joint or choose a different outcome measure, such as time (in seconds) to transfer out of a chair, distance from fingertips to floor (cm), pulse, or even blood pressure. You should select an outcome measure that you typically use in your clinic. Parenthetically, running more than 10 patients would be desirable and the needed sample size could be estimated using power analysis.

Collecting Data

Instructions. Measure right shoulder abduction using the same goniometer for 10 patients on two separate occasions. There should be no intervention for the right shoulder between occasions. The first set of measurements might represent a Monday measurement of right shoulder abduction for 10 patients taken during an initial evaluation, and the second set, Wednesday measurements for the same 10 patients before the initiation of treatment (Figure 23-1). Take measurements in the manner you typically do in the clinic. Make sure your measurements are not influenced by knowledge of previous measurements.

Caution. If the patients have similar or normal shoulder abduction ranges (e.g., scores clustering between 165 and 180 degrees), analysis may not yield the true measure of reliability. If this is the case, choose a measure that provides a fuller range of possible scores (see Chapter 12).

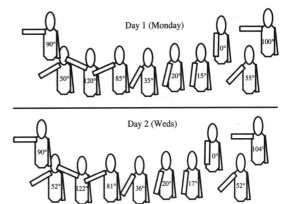

Figure 23-1.   Intrarater reliability of measurement of shoulder abduction range of motion after each patient is measured twice (Monday and Wednesday) by the same clinician and shows how well each patient's shoulder range corresponds for the 2 days.

Analysis of the Data

Conduct a Correlational Analysis

STEP 1. ENTER DATA ONTO A SPREADSHEET.   Notes: statistical assumptions for correlation analysis must first be satisfied (see Chapter 20). In this example, the α level has been set at .05. The first step in examining the data is to enter them into an SPSS spreadsheet (see Chapter 10).

1. Open SPSS.
2. Go to FILE.
3. Select NEW FILE. Enter your data below in two columns. The first column represents range of motion on Monday, and the second represents range of motion on Wednesday. There should be 10 entries in each column.

   Column 1 (VAR00001): 90, 50, 120, 85, 35, 20, 15, 0, 55, 100
   Column 2 (VAR00001): 95, 52, 122, 81, 36, 20, 17, 0, 52, 104

4. Go to FILE.
5. Select PRINT. Print the spreadsheet and compare the accuracy of entries with the data, because errors in entry can occur.

STEP 2. CONDUCT A CORRELATIONAL ANALYSIS

1. In SPSS, go to ANALYZE.
2. Select CORRELATE.
3. Select BIVARIATE. Highlight the two variables (on the left side of the screen), and use the arrow button to move the variable (VAR00001 and VAR00002) into the variable box on the right side of the screen.
4. Click on Pearson box.
5. Click on two-tailed test.
6. Click on OK. This starts the analysis.

7. The output should read as follows:

Pearson Correlation   .998
Sig. (2-tailed)   000
N   10

INTERPRETATION.   The Pearson correlation (r value) is .99 (in this example), which indicates an excellent (almost perfect) positive correspondence between the Monday and the Wednesday measurements. That is, intrarater reliability is excellent. Any r value greater than .90 would be acceptable reliability for this clinical measure.[2] If the r value is less than .90, you should reflect on why your measurements are less consistent. Perhaps they can be improved if you standardize your measurement technique so that you measure each patient the same way.

The significance level (Sig) of 000 does not mean zero significance. It indicates a P value less than .0005 for SPSS software. That is, the value is statistically significant; this relationship would occur by chance fewer than 5 times in 10,000.[3] In other words, the relationship probably did not occur by chance.

N indicates that there were 10 pairs of scores in your analysis.

To obtain a visual display of the association (recommended), follow the steps in Chapter 12 to display a scatter plot. A linear pattern (straight line) of the data suggests a strong association.

Is There Agreement between the First and Second Sets of Scores?   You can determine how well your first measurements agree with your second measurements. To do this, use the ICC.

1. In SPSS, go to ANALYZE.
2. Select SCALE.
3. Select RELIABILITY ANALYSIS.
4. Select and move the two variables (Monday and Wednesday measurements) into the box.
5. Click on STATISTICS BOX.
6. Click on INTRACLASS CORRELATION COEFFICIENT. Review Chapter 12 for choice and interpretation of ICC.
7. For ICC (2,1), select TWO-WAY RANDOM model and ABSOLUTE AGREEMENT.
8. For ICC (3,1), select TWO-WAY MIXED model and CONSISTENCY.
9. Click on OK.
10. Look at the results (called the *output* of the computer analysis). The ICC value in the output can be identified under *Single Measure Intraclass Correlation*. The P value can be identified under *Sig. = .*
11. Review Chapter 12 if you are not clear how to interpret the results of the analysis.

ESTABLISHING INTERRATER RELIABILITY

If your clinic has different therapists taking measurements of the same patient, establishing interrater reliability makes sense. Interrater reliability often is not as good as intrarater reliability. In other words, clinicians generally are capable of agreeing with themselves more than they are with others. This lack of agreement is analogous to two clinicians identifying different problems or treatment recommendations for the same patient—a not uncommon situation.

Collecting Data

Perhaps you see patients on Mondays and another clinician sees the same patients on Wednesdays. The first set of measurements represents *your* Monday measurement of right shoulder abduction for 10 patients. The second set of measurements is those obtained for the same 10 patients on Wednesday by *the other clinician*.

Analyzing the Data

Conduct a Correlational Analysis.   Repeat the procedures described for intrarater reliability. The only difference in the procedure is that a different clinician has taken the second set of measurements.

STEP 1. ENTER THE DATA

1. Enter the following data in two columns. The first column represents Monday range of motion recorded by you, and the second column represents Wednesday range of motion recorded by the other clinician. There should be 10 entries in each column.

   Column 1 (VAR00001): 90, 50, 120, 85, 35, 20, 15, 0, 55, 100
   Column 2 (VAR00001): 80, 70, 130, 95, 38, 24, 21, 0, 48, 100

2. Go to FILE.
3. Select PRINT. Print the spreadsheet and compare the accuracy of entries with the data, because errors in entry can occur.

STEP 2. CONDUCT A CORRELATIONAL ANALYSIS IN SPSS

1. Go to ANALYZE.
2. Select CORRELATE.
3. Select BIVARIATE.
4. Highlight the two variables (on the left side of the screen), and use the arrow button to move the variable (VAR00001 and VAR00002) into the variable box on the right side of the screen.
5. Click on Pearson box.
6. Click on two-tailed test.
7. Click on OK. This starts the analysis.
8. The output should read as follows:

   Pearson Correlation   .977
   Sig. (2-tailed)   000
   N   10

INTERPRETATION OF INTERRATER RELIABILITY.   The Pearson correlation (r value) is .97, which indicates an excellent (almost perfect) positive correspondence between the two clinicians. That is, interrater reliability is excellent. For this example, interrater reliability is only slightly less than intrarater reliability. Any value greater than .90 would be acceptable reliability for this clinical measure.[2] For values less than .90, you should reflect on why your measurements are less consistent. Perhaps they can be improved if you standardize your measurement technique or train clinicians so that each applies the same technique to assess joint range.

The significance level (Sig) of 000 does not mean zero significance. It indicates that the *P* value is less than .0005. It is statistically significant, and this relationship would have occurred by chance fewer than 5 times in 10,000. The relationship probably did not occur by chance.

N indicates that there were 10 pairs of scores in your analysis, that is, 10 patients.

It is good practice to examine the scatter plot.

Agreement between Two Clinicians: Intraclass Correlation Coefficient.   You can also determine the ICC (described earlier) to determine how well measurements of the two clinicians agree.

SUMMARY

Clinicians should begin to see the value of establishing reliability—intrarater and interrater—in the clinic with tools such as goniometers for documentation, case reports, quality assurance procedures, and research endeavors. If measurements are not consistently taken, how do you, the patient, other health care practitioners, insurance companies, or even the courts know whether changes in measurements are attributed to real changes in the patient or simply error (inconsistency) in taking measurements?

WRITING A CASE REPORT

A case report gives the clinician the opportunity to report unusual phenomenon, typically in one patient, and thus contribute to the body of knowledge. A case can represent an individual or an institution, and an author can report a series of cases (called a *case series*). The first two sections of this chapter (the literature, participating in a journal club reviewing, and establishing reliability) lay the foundation for writing a case report. The following elements usually are included in a case report.

BACKGROUND

The literature provides background information on a problem. Literature reviews and participation in journal clubs can help familiarize clinicians with what has been reported in the field so they can identify new cases (see Chapters 4, 21, and 22).

The Purpose or Problem

For a case report, all that is needed is an unusual or unique observation in clinical practice (see Chapters 4 and 7). Case reports typically evolve out of a clinician's need to aid a patient.[4]

Example

You are treating a patient with a diagnosis of a "right frozen shoulder" who is unable to raise his right arm over his head. You give the patient a weight but then leave him for 5 minutes so that you can answer the telephone. When you return, the patient is leaning against a table and rocking his torso so that his right hand, which was holding the weight, hangs down and gently swings back and forth as a pendulum does. The patient reports that it feels like a "good, relaxing stretch." When you start to exercise the patient's right arm, you notice, to your amazement, that the patient can now raise his arm 35 degrees more than he could before you left the room. Because you believe this observation is important and has not been previously reported in the literature, you decide to write a case report. (Although this is a fictitious story about Codman's exercise, it is instructive in describing one way a case report can originate.)

PATIENT DESCRIPTION

Describe the patient in sufficient detail. Patients who possess similar characteristics can then be identified and targeted in future studies. For example, the description in 1981 by Hymes et al.[5] of a group of young men who had a form of cancer not typical for that age group was important in what came to be known as AIDS.

Information about the patient includes age; sex; ethnicity; race; diagnosis; prognosis; previous treatments; medical history; results of past and current diagnostic investigations, such as magnetic resonance imaging, computed tomography, and laboratory tests; medications; psychological tests; clinical and functional assessment (a separate section entitled "Examination" is often included in case reports); employment status; social situation; and current intervention if any. Including a figure of the patient or lesion (photographs, radiographs, MRI) can be helpful in illustrating the problem or pathology, if the patient has given consent to do so.

The examination gives the reader information about the patient's "current" condition during the clinician's first encounter with the patient. This information can be conveyed through a clinical assessment section (i.e., impairments: strength, range of motion, sensation, balance, endurance, posture) and a functional assessment section (i.e., gait, transfers, bed mobility, dressing, eating, grooming, changing money, ability to work).

INSTRUMENTS

Case reports include carefully recorded, unbiased observations.[4] Any measuring instruments used should be described in sufficient detail (name, model number, and name and location of manufacturer) because the author of the report may rely on these instruments in making observations. A photograph or illustration of the instrument is helpful to readers if the instrument is uncommon or newly developed.

Information on the validity of the measuring instrument can be included so that readers know what it is supposed to measure and perhaps how accurately it performs compared to a standard (criterion validity; see Chapter 9).

Information on the reliability of the measuring instrument should be included. Measuring instruments have to be reliable because they are used for repeated assessments of patients. Because clinicians repeatedly measure patients over time to indicate progress, it makes sense to establish reliability of measurements, *even for a case report.* If only one clinician had taken all measurements for a case, establishing intrarater reliability is desirable. If two or more clinicians had taken measurements, establishing interrater reliability is desirable.

Reliability and validity are not always reported in case reports, perhaps because case reports are not used to demonstrate causality. Nevertheless, valid tools can strengthen the credibility of your observations of the patient because your measurements affect your observations and the interpretation.[4] Valid and reliable measures are even more crucial if you use single-subject or experimental designs in the future.

COURSE OF TREATMENT

The events that inspire a case report usually lack the strictly controlled rigor of an experiment. The author has had no plan to manipulate or intentionally elicit an observation for research.[4] Hopefully all events in patient care had been meticulously recorded. Typically, these observations and interventions are entered into the medical chart. The more detailed the entries, the better is the report—you are writing a detailed story about this unique observation. For example, "on week one, the patient received ultrasound treatment three times a week for 10 minutes at 1.5 W/cm^2 over the anterior right shoulder. On week 2 through 4 . . . ." If observations are not documented in a timely manner, memory may fade, and important evidence can be lost.

Example

For a patient with a pressure ulcer associated with wheelchair use, documenting cushion type, number of hours spent sitting, activity level (ability to weight shift off the ulcer), sensation, climate, and wheelchair fit may be important information.[6]

OUTCOME/RESULTS

A case report does not require sophisticated statistical analyses (N = 1). Instead, a description of performance or behavior with raw scores, percentages, means and standard deviations, the coefficient of variation, and error scores is adequate.

Analysis

A few descriptive analyses are as follows.

Raw Scores. Raw scores (individual original scores) can be reported for one point in time or over time. Examples of raw scores include 10 degrees of knee flexion measured with a goniometer, 30 seconds standing on one foot measured with a stop watch, 2.5-cm pressure ulcer measured with a tape measure, 15 pounds (6.75 kg) of grip strength measured with a dynamometer, and a 6-day hospital stay.

Example

The pressure ulcer decreased in diameter from 2.5 cm in January to 2.0 cm in February and 0.3 cm in March 2000. (Each measurement, taken once, is a raw score.)

Percentage. The percentage of patient's successful performances is a quotient of the number of times the patient accomplishes a task and the total number of attempts multiplied by 100 ([Number of successes ÷ Total number of trials] × 100).[7] How do I calculate it?

Example: Getting Out of a Chair

Trial 1 successful
Trial 2 successful
Trial 3 successful
Trial 4 not successful
Trial 5 successful
Trial 6 successful
Trial 7 not successful
Trial 8 successful
Trial 9 successful
Trial 10 not successful

Seven of 10 trials are successful, so

Percentage = (Successful trials ÷ All trials) × 100
7/10 × 100 = .7 × 100 = 70%

At initial evaluation, the patient can stand from sitting 70% of the time. That is, he was able to stand 7 times successfully out of 10 attempts.

Mean Value and Standard Deviation. The mean, the average of several raw scores, and the standard deviation, a measure of variability, are discussed at length in Chapter 10. The advantage of taking an average is that it is a better estimate of the true value of something than is any individual score. The mean and standard deviation can be reported for one point in time or over time.

Example

The patient's ability to stand unsupported in 10 trials improved on average from 5 seconds (2 SD) at initial evaluation to 120 seconds (20 SD) at discharge.

Coefficient of Variation. The coefficient of variation (CV) is used to measure the *relative variability* in a phenomenon. The CV is easily calculated by dividing the standard deviation by the mean (SD/Mean) and then multiplying by 100 to obtain a percentage of variation.[2] The CV is useful for comparing variability of different samples.

Example

What is the consistency of a clinician's force production of spinal mobilization in 10 trials after a training session. How do I calculate it?

Trial	Raw Score (pounds)
1	40
2	44
3	34
4	41
5	45
6	39
7	42
8	38
9	42
10	37

First calculate the mean (Sum of scores ÷ Number of scores) and standard deviation using SPSS, Excel, or equivalent software (see Chapter 10).

Mean = 3.33
SD = 40.20
CV = (SD ÷ Mean) × 100 = 3.33/40.20 × 100
   = .08 × 100 = 8%

Spinal mobilization forces were more consistent after training. The CV decreased from 16% before training to 8% after training.

Absolute Error.   Absolute error provides a general measure of error when the direction of error is not important. Absolute error can be derived when the patient has a target performance and there is a way of measuring the amount of error that the patient deviates from that target.

Absolute error is calculated by means of subtracting the desired criterion target from each actual performance for each trial, taking the absolute value of each difference score so there are no negative scores, summing these absolute difference scores, and dividing this sum by the number of trials. The result is mean or average absolute error value. It is always positive.[8] How do I calculate it? (Chapter 9 describes absolute error for individual scores.)

Trial	Raw Score (pounds)	Criterion Target 40 Pounds	Difference Score
1	40	–40	0
2	44	–40	+4
3	34	–40	–6
4	41	–40	+1
5	45	–40	+5
6	39	–40	–1
7	42	–40	+2
8	38	–40	–2
9	42	–40	+2
10	37	–40	–3
			26

The sum of absolute difference score is 26. (The scores are added without regard to sign.)

Absolute error = Sum of absolute difference scores
   ÷ Number of scores = 26/10 = 2.6 pounds.

After a training program, the clinician's ability to match the desired mobilization force to a target force improved. His absolute error decreased from 7.5 pounds to 2.6 pounds (3.4 kg to 1.2 kg) after training.

Constant Error.   Constant error provides a measure of bias (overshooting or undershooting error) of a target and therefore is used to measure both *directions of error* and the amount of error. It is derived by means of subtracting the desired criterion target from each actual performance for each trial, summing these difference scores, which may be positive or negative, and then dividing this sum by the number of trials.[8] The resulting score, which is averaged, may be positive, indicating overshooting or positive bias, or negative, indicating undershooting or negative bias. Patients who are tentative or cautious may undershoot targets. (Chapter 9 reviews constant error for individual scores.) How do I calculate it?

Trial	Raw Score (pounds)	Criterion Target 40 Pounds	Difference Score
1	40	–40	0
2	44	–40	+4
3	34	–40	–6
4	41	–40	+1
5	45	–40	+5
6	39	–40	–1
7	42	–40	+2
8	38	–40	–2
9	42	–40	+2
10	37	–40	–3
			+2

The sum of difference score is +2.

Constant error = Sum of difference scores
   ÷ Number of scores = +2/10 = +0.2 pounds (+90 g).

The clinician tended to slightly overshoot the target force after training. His constant error was +0.2 pounds (+90 g).

Figures

Graphs give data a sense of pattern. The data in the last example can be presented visually with different types of graphs—line graphs, bar graphs, and box-and-whisker plots. For presentations and publication, these graphs can be constructed easily with spreadsheet software such as Powerpoint, Excel, or SPSS.

Line graphs are an excellent way to display an outcome over time (e.g., over a period of seconds, minutes, hours, days, or weeks). The time period is located on the horizontal (*x*) axis, and the outcome measure is located on the vertical (*y*) axis. For example, line graphs can illustrate improvements in skill level (reduced absolute error performance) or attainment of range of motion over time (Figure 23-2).

Bar graphs display performance under different conditions, each bar representing a different condition, treatment, skill, or category. For example, bar graphs can indicate improvement in range of motion at baseline and at time of discharge (Figure 23-3A). Bar graphs also can illustrate amount of time to don different articles of clothing (Figure 23-3B).

Histograms and box-and-whisker plots can illustrate the distribution (variability) of raw scores in a performance (see Figures 10-9 and 10-10).

Tables

Tables are useful for displaying detailed information including summary scores, such as means, standard deviations, and *r* values.

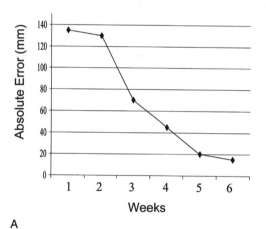

A

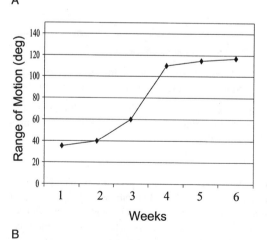

B

Figure 23-2.   Line graphs are useful for displaying performance over time. (**A**) Amount of absolute error in aiming for a target (elevator button) over time. (**B**) Range of motion measurements over time.

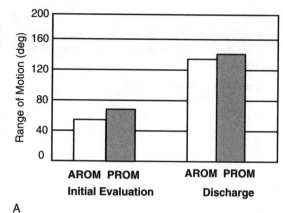

A

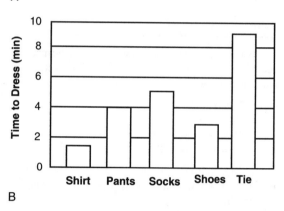

B

Figure 23-3.   Bar graphs are useful at displaying performance under different conditions. (**A**) Amount of shoulder range of motion at initial evaluation and at discharge. *AROM,* Active range of motion; *PROM,* passive range of motion. (**B**) Amount of time to don different articles of clothing.

DISCUSSION AND CONCLUSIONS OF A CASE REPORT

One of the chief goals of reporting cases is to *generate hypotheses*. The discussion should be used to interpret data and propose hypotheses (predictions), which can be confirmed in another study with a correlational or experimental design.[4] The intent of authors of case reports is to explore, infer, and discover rather than to confirm, deduce, or prove.

The author should indicate the unique contribution of the report to the literature, how the report relates to other reports in the literature if there are any (i.e., agree or not in agreement with previous findings), and suggest the next step in research. That next step may be to test the hypothesis generated in the case.[4] For example, one hypothesis generated from the Codman's exercise case report (described earlier) may be that "distraction of the shoulder joint caused by holding a weight improves shoulder abduction among persons with frozen shoulders." A follow-up experiment that manipulates the variable *weight* can test this hypothesis.

Authors need to be careful what they conclude in case reports. Case reports cannot demonstrate causality or associations or argue for adoption of a new treatment approach. They also cannot generalize the findings for one person to an entire population of similar patients, because the report is limited to only one patient (N = 1).[4] A case report should not read, "This treatment was the cause" (that is, there were no other contributing factors), "This treatment should now be implemented in practice," or "All patients similar to this patient will respond the same way."

A case report is only the first step in research, not the last. It is an excellent design for clinicians to *discover* but not to prove.

SHARING KNOWLEDGE

Your case will not add to the body of knowledge unless it is shared with others. Three traditions exist for sharing knowledge in science—poster presentation, platform presentation, and journal article. The Internet, for example a home page, is another way to share information but is not subject to peer review except for peer-reviewed online journals.

POSTER PRESENTATIONS

A low-stress first step in sharing information about a case is to submit it as a poster presentation at a professional conference. A poster is a written description of the report and often is presented with photographs, illustrations, and graphs. The author attaches the written materials to a 4-foot by 8-foot corkboard and stands by the poster for a designated time during the conference to discuss the work with others who may show interest.

Applications for poster presentations typically are found in an association's professional journal. Follow the instructions on the application for writing an abstract of the case. If the abstract is accepted, additional information on guidelines for making the poster will follow. If they do not, request them. One advantage of poster presentations is interaction with colleagues. Another is that the abstract may be published in the journal.

PLATFORM PRESENTATIONS

A platform presentation involves formally addressing an audience about a study. The talk usually lasts between 10 to 15 minutes and is followed by questions from the audience. Platform presentation does not usually produce the helpful feedback that poster presentations do. Nevertheless, platform presentation is a time-honored tradition in science.[2] It is a good choice if the work can be better

communicated through slides or transparencies with formal commentary rather than through a poster with informal commentary. The preference for a platform presentation can be indicated on the conference application. As for a poster, the abstract of a platform presentation may be published in the association's journal.

Suggestions for Slide Presentations

- Summarize slides. Do not read verbatim from slides; the audience can read.
- Do not crowd the slide with too many lines. No more than six lines is the guideline.[2]
- Choose a simple font and make the type large enough so the audience can read the slide from the back of the room.[2]
- Do not use irritating background or difficult-to-see foreground colors. A dark blue background with orange or white letters is a good choice.

If you are giving a platform presentation (you must thrive on stress), time and practice the talk until it is perfect, and then practice again. On the day of the presentation, go to the presentation room early and check to make sure all the equipment—projectors, microphone, laser pointer, house lights—works properly before you get on stage.

PUBLICATION

The third way to share information is to submit your case as a manuscript for publication in a peer-reviewed journal. Submission of a manuscript is the next logical step after a poster or platform presentation. Guidelines for submitting manuscripts can be found in each journal. It is crucial that you know the readership of the journal; the manuscript is likely to be rejected if the report does not match the goals and interests of the journal and its readers. For example, do not submit a rehabilitation medicine report to a general medical journal unless the topic has broad appeal. Your work must be critically reviewed and accepted by your peers (called *peer review*) before it is accepted for publication. The advantage of publication of an article in a journal is permanent exposure of your peer-reviewed work to a large audience. Your publication also is likely to be indexed, for example, in the *Index Medicus* and MEDLINE, for search by other researchers.

Suggestion for Preparing for Publication

Revise, revise, revise: For scientific writing, you need to say what you mean clearly, concisely, without repetition, with the fewest number of pages, and with the least amount of ink. This typically requires multiple revisions of the manuscript.

SUMMARY

A case report is an important first step in the research process because it can often lead to important new questions that can later be answered with more sophisticated research designs. Clinicians, because of their access to patients, are in a unique position to contribute to this process by writing and presenting case reports.

REFERENCES

1. Alguire PC. A review of journal clubs in postgraduate medical education. *J Gen Intern Med.* 1998;13:347–353.
2. Portney LG, Watkins MP. *Foundations of Clinical Research: Applications to Practice.* Upper Saddle River, N.J.: Prentice Hall; 2000.
3. Einspruch EL. *An Introductory Guide to SPSS for Windows.* Thousand Oaks, Calif: Sage Publications; 1998.
4. Bolgar H. The case study method. In: Wolman BB, ed. *Handbook of Clinical Psychology.* New York: McGraw-Hill; 1965:28–39.
5. Hymes KB, Cheung T, Greene JB, et al. Kaposi's sarcoma in homosexual men: a report of eight cases. *Lancet.* 1981;2:598–600.
6. Batavia M, Batavia AI. Pressure ulcer in a man with tetraplegia and a poorly fitting wheelchair: a case report with clinical and policy implication. *Spinal Cord.* 1999;37:141.
7. Burrell B. *Merriam-Webster's Guide to Everyday Math: A Home and Business Reference.* Springfield, Mass: Merriam-Webster; 1998.
8. Magill RA. *Motor Learning: Concepts and Applications.* 4th ed. Madison, Wis: WCB Brown & Benchmark; 1993.

24

Just for Graduate Students

This chapter discusses (1) desirable characteristics of a graduate student and (2) a survival list to enhance the graduate experience or at least make it far less miserable. By *graduate student,* I am referring primarily to postprofessional graduate students who are required to produce a substantial research project, at either the masters or the doctoral level.

DESIRABLE CHARACTERISTICS OF A GRADUATE STUDENT

ATTITUDE: IT IS A JOURNEY

The joy of being a graduate student comes when you realize that you have embarked on a unique journey—such as the yellow brick road in the Land of Oz—with many adventures along the way. Unlike the yellow brick road, the trail you blaze is your own. Some of the adventures have a disappointing outcome, but these make the successful outcomes all the more gratifying. Think of graduate school as a process whereby you solve a series of problems in the ultimate pursuit of creating knowledge. Enjoy the journey.

CURIOSITY

Curiosity is difficult if not impossible to teach and yet may not be necessary to learn. Human beings are innately curious.[1] If you are in a research area that does not pique your interest, find one that will.

SCHOLARLY BEHAVIOR

Becoming a scholar means presenting ideas in a civilized, unbiased, and unemotional way with the goal of learning and contributing to knowledge rather than proving one's point.

JACK OF ALL TRADES AND MASTER OF ONE: ON BECOMING A RENAISSANCE PERSON

To successfully complete a thesis or dissertation, graduate students may need to develop many new skills. For example, they may need to think as an inventor, write as an author, communicate as a diplomat, repair equipment as a machinist, compute as a statistician, and recruit subjects as an administrator. In addition to all this, a graduate student needs to become an expert in one area of research. In short, the graduate experience provides the wonderful opportunity to grow as a human being. It should be welcomed as a good thing.

INDEPENDENT WORKER

Graduate students do independent work. It is unacceptable to run to the committee with every problem before attempting to solve it. Taking credit for someone else's idea or having someone do the work is far worse. For example, stating in an oral defense that "My statistician told me to do it that way" is a death sentence. Even if they consult with experts, graduate students are ultimately responsible for understanding and conducting every facet of their studies. In short, do your own work and view problems as simply part of the learning process. You are being trained to solve problems. Overcoming these obstacles on your own can be one of the most gratifying experiences in graduate school and life.

PERSEVERANCE

Perseverance is necessary for graduate students. There are many opportunities for failure. For example, the research question may have to be abandoned, subject recruitment may be slow, equipment may break down, and data may be more difficult to interpret than first anticipated.

Attempts at publishing may be plagued by rejection. None of this is unusual. If any of it happens to you, you are in excellent company. The good news is, perseverance usually is rewarded.

SURVIVAL LIST FOR GRADUATE STUDENTS

START THINKING ABOUT A QUESTION EARLY

For doctoral students, identifying an original question is a difficult task and may take a year or longer. Masters students, who may not be required to conduct original research, can consider replicating previously published studies. Replication can confirm that previous findings are reliable and not simply due to chance. Replication also is needed in health-related research, in which sample sizes tend to be small (A. McDonough, oral communication, October 1999). Regardless of your goals, start thinking about a question early.

CHOOSE YOUR COMMITTEE WISELY

Choose committee members who can positively contribute their expertise to your project. You should also feel comfortable working with them. For example, if you are a behaviorist and the committee is made up of cognitive psychologists, you may be inviting disaster. If you like qualitative research and want to conduct interviews, and your committee is made up of quantitative experimentalists who use electromyography and force plates, you may be a masochist. Ask the chair of your committee, once selected, for his or her suggestions for other members. It is ideal that the committee members have a good working relationship.

LEARN HOW TO WORK WITH YOUR COMMITTEE AND PEOPLE IN GENERAL

All committee members work differently. Some members like to have periodic meetings, whereas others prefer to communicate by e-mail or telephone. Committee members may have their own preferences about the number of chapters they want to read at one time and the amount of time they need to review your work. Simply ask each member how he or she prefers to work with you.

Most important is never to play one committee member against another, as by saying "She told me to do it this way." Weigh all input from each member, be diplomatic, and suggest a course of action based on evidence, such as literature or pilot work. A confident, well-thought-out plan usually is welcomed by all.

ACCEPT CONSTRUCTIVE CRITICISM

Nothing is more disappointing than watching an arrogant student ignore faculty suggestions and constructive criticism when the student is clearly clueless about his or her own study. Show gratitude, humility, and receptiveness to constructive criticism. The committee members know the ropes and can help you.

KEEP IN TOUCH

Keep your committee or advisor informed about your progress. Do not disappear for months or years then reappear out of nowhere and expect everyone to drop what he or she is doing so you can make a deadline.

BE REALISTIC

Things take longer than you think. Do not say to your committee in the late spring that you expect to obtain institutional review board approval by June, collect data in the summer, and graduate in the fall if you do not yet have a well-formulated question. You are kidding yourself. Some things cannot be rushed; a research proposal is one of them.

RESPOND TO QUESTIONS

At meetings with committee members or advisors, or in a colloquium, respond to questions about your study in a scholarly, unemotional manner. Audiotaping or videotaping the meeting if all agree may be a useful teaching aid to hear or see how you behave under pressure.

A useful technique is to repeat the question. There are four advantages to this. First, if the question upsets you emotionally, repeating it buys you a few moments to cool off. Second, repeating the question provides time for you to think about the question. Third, you confirm whether you heard the question correctly. Fourth, others in the audience may not have heard the question.

SURROUND YOURSELF WITH SUPPORTIVE PEOPLE

Graduate work can seem isolating. Friends and family members may not understand what you are going through. It is therefore important to have a support group or friends who are willing to lend an ear because you will no doubt be frustrated at times.

KNOW YOUR MOTIVATION FOR OBTAINING A DOCTORATE

If you are in graduate school to obtain a doctorate, such as doctor of philosophy or doctor of education, understand what motivates you to pursue this challenging degree. Certainly the degree trains you to conduct research, enables you to pursue teaching, and can transport you on a personal journey of human growth. If, however, the honest reason is to achieve some notion of status, the journey can be frustrating, painful, costly, and ultimately unsuccessful.

REFERENCE

1. Hazen RM, Trefil J. *Science Matters: Achieving Scientific Literacy.* New York: Doubleday, 1991.

25

The Future: A Final Word . . .
or Two . . . or Three

RESEARCHER AND CLINICIAN COLLABORATION

The goal of this book is to enhance understanding and appreciation of clinical research. Graduate students and clinicians training to become researchers should begin to see the overall perspective in planning a study. Some may catch the research "bug" and engage in a lifelong career of research. Those involved primarily in patient care may become better consumers of the literature and may want to take the first steps in research, such as case reporting. My hope is that researchers and clinicians will collaborate on research projects more in the future. Why? So we can help patients by using our growing knowledge base.

THE CLINICIAN'S DILEMMA

Clinicians need to know how important they are to the research community and growing knowledge base. Clinicians ask clinically important questions, have access to the patient populations needed to answer those questions, and have the necessary credentials and expertise to administer relevant treatments. Unfortunately, clinicians do not have the luxury of conducting research because administration does not always provide time for these activities unless they are quality assurance activities.

THE RESEARCHER'S DILEMMA

Researchers have the training, time, and motivation, such as the pressure of making tenure, to design a study, collect data, analyze results, and compile the findings for publication. They are trained to convert clinically important questions into questions that can be answered with the scientific method. Unfortunately, researchers do not always have

access to populations, funding, or the assistance to conduct studies, for example to administer treatments.

A POSSIBLE SOLUTION

If researchers and clinicians who have common patient concerns can meet (even outside work), draw on each other's strengths, and conduct research projects together, our knowledge base can grow substantially from a pebble to a mountain.

RESEARCH: A WORK IN PROGRESS

Research is a human endeavor, and as such it is subject to error (see Appendix B). Over the long run, replication of findings by others is the best means to guard against the many potential errors in research. Thus, a research project should be considered a work in progress rather than the final word on a problem.

KEEPING RESEARCH IN PERSPECTIVE

It may be insightful to place research in proper perspective. The following adage has been adapted from Hazen and Trefil.[1(p278)]

> We probe the world, using science
> Search for its meaning, with philosophy
> And appreciate it, through the arts.

REFERENCE

1. Hazen RM, Trefil J. *Science Matters: Achieving Scientific Literacy*. New York: Doubleday, 1991.

Appendix A
Resources

BOOKS ON SEARCHING THE INTERNET

Berinstein P. *Finding Statistics Online: How to Locate the Elusive Numbers You Need.* Medford, N.J.: Information Today; 1998.

Davis JB. *Health and Medicine on the Internet: Annual Guide to the World Wide Web.* Los Angeles: Health Information Press; 1997.

Griffin AD. *Directory of Internet Sources for Health Professional.* Albany, N.Y.: Delmar Publishers; 1999.

Maxwell B. *How to Find Health Information on the Internet.* Washington, DC: Congressional Quarterly; 1998.

Maxwell B. *How to Access the Federal Government on the Internet.* 4th ed. Washington D.C.: Congressional Quarterly; 1999.

Notess GR. *Government Information on the Internet.* 2nd ed. Lanham, Md: Bernan Press; 1998.

Schlein AM. Find It Online: The Complete Guide to Online Research. Tempe, Ariz: Facts on Demand; 1999. [Comment: This is a great resource for getting up to speed with searches on the Internet. It includes examples of searches.]

GRANT INFORMATION FOR FUNDING RESEARCH

Annual Register of Grant Support: A Directory of Funding Sources. 3rd ed. New Providence, N.J.: RR Bowker; 1998.

Directory of Biomedical and Health Care Grants 2000. 14th ed. Phoenix: Oryx Press; 1999. [Comment: Includes more than 4000 human health and biomedical funding programs.]

STYLE MANUALS FOR PUBLISHING IN JOURNALS

American Medical Association Manual of Style: A Guide for Authors and Editors. 9th ed. Baltimore: Williams & Wilkins; 1998.

The Chicago Manual of Style. 14th ed. Chicago: University of Chicago Press; 1993.

Publication Manual of the American Psychological Association. 4th ed. Washington, DC: American Psychological Association; 1994.

BOOKS ON RESEARCH DESIGNS AND METHODS

Campbell DT, Stanley JC. *Experimental and Quasi-experimental Designs for Research.* Boston: Houghton Mifflin; 1963. [Comment: A classic on experimental and quasi-experimental research designs.]

Kirk RE. *Experimental Design: Procedures for the Behavioral Sciences.* Monterey, Calif: Brooks/Cole; 1982.

Light RJ, Singer JD, Willett JB. *By Design: Planning Research on Higher Education.* Cambridge, Mass: Harvard University Press; 1990. [Comment: This is a well-written and practical approach to dealing with design issues in educational research.]

Maddox T, ed. Tests: *A Comprehensive Reference for Assessments in Psychology, Education, and Business.* 4th ed. Austin, Tex: Pro-ed; 1997.

McDonough AL. *LabVIEW: Data Acquisition and Analysis for the Movement Sciences.* Upper Saddle River, N.J.: Prentice Hall; 2000. [Comment: Teaches you how to write your own data collection programs using LabVIEW to collect and analyze human performance data. For information on courses, contact: http://www.nyu.edu/classes/mcdonough/m&eiii.htm.]

Portney LG, Watkins MP. *Foundations of Clinical Research: Applications to Practice.* Upper Saddle River, N.J.: Prentice Hall, 2000. [Comment: A good resource for clinical research, particularly for physical rehabilitation specialists.]

BOOKS ON STATISTICS AND MATH

Burrell B. *Merriam-Webster's Guide to Everyday Math: A Home and Business Reference.* Springfield, Mass: Merriam-Webster; 1998. [Comment: An easy to read, practical, and informative guide to math.]

Hartwig F, Dearing BE. *Exploratory Data Analysis.* Beverly Hills, Calif: Sage Publications; 1978. [Comment: A lucid description of descriptive statistics and the importance of examining data graphically.]

Munro BH. *Statistical Methods for Health Care Research.* 4th ed. Philadelphia: Lippincott Williams & Wilkins; 2000. [Comment: An instructive guide to understanding and interpreting statistics.]

Schroeder LD, Sjoquist DL, Stephan PE. *Understanding Regression Analysis: An Introductory Guide.* Newbury Park, Calif: Sage Publications; 1986. [Comment: An easy to read book on regression.]

BOOKS ON SCIENCE

Beveridge WIB. *The Art of Scientific Investigation.* 3rd ed. New York: Vintage Books; 1957. [Comment: A classic book on discoveries in science.]

Hazen RM, Trefil J. *Science Matters: Achieving Scientific Literacy.* New York: Doubleday; 1991. [Comment: One of the best summaries of principles in science.]

HEALTH INFORMATION

Directories of Consumer Health Information on the Internet.
- Hardin Meta Directory of Internet Health Sources. Available at: http://www.lib.uiowa.edu/hardin/md/index.html.
- Healthfinder. Available at: http://www.healthfinder.gov.

CONTACTING INDUSTRIES FOR MATERIALS

Medical Device Register. 19th ed. Montvale, N.J.: Medical Economics; 1999.

Thomas Register of American Manufacturers. Available at: http://www.thomasregister.com.

Appendix B
List of Potential Biases in Research

The following material is reprinted from Sackett DL. Bias in analytic research. *J Chron Dis*. 1979;32:60–63 (appendix). Used with permission.

A CATALOG OF BIASES

DEFINITION OF BIAS

"Any process at any stage of inference that tends to produce results or conclusions that differ systematically from the truth." (Adapted from Murphy. *The Logic of Medicine*. Baltimore: Johns Hopkins University Press; 1976.)

STAGES OF RESEARCH IN WHICH BIAS CAN OCCUR

An outline of the catalog.

(1) In *reading-up* on the field.
(2) In specifying and selecting the study *sample*.
(3) In *executing* the experimental *manoeuvre* (or exposure).
(4) In *measuring* exposures and outcomes.
(5) In *analyzing* the data.
(6) In *interpreting* the analysis.
(7) In *publishing* the results [and back to (1)].

THE CATALOG

Each bias is defined and followed by an example.

(1) In *reading-up* on the field:
(a) *The biases of rhetoric*. Any of several techniques used to convince the reader without appealing to reason, e.g. Good IJ: a classification of fallacious arguments and interpretations. *Technometrics*. 4: 125–132, 1962.
(b) *The all's well literature bias*. Scientific or professional societies may publish reports or editorials that omit or play down controversies or disparate results, e.g. the debate on "control" and the complications of diabetes, well shown in editorials in the *New Engl J Med* 294: 1004, 1976 and 296: 1228–1229, 1977.
(c) *One-sided reference bias*. Authors may restrict their references to only those works that support their position: a literature review with a single starting point risks confinement to a single side of the issues, e.g. Platt and Pickering on the inheritance of hypertension; Hamilton, Pickering et al.: *Clin Sci*. 24: 91–108, 1963; Platt: *Lancet* 1: 899–904, 1963.
(d) *Positive results bias*. Authors are more likely to submit, and editors accept, positive than null results, e.g. multiple personal experiences.
(e) *Hot stuff bias*. When a topic is hot, neither investigation no editors may be able to resist the temptation to publish additional results, no matter how preliminary or shaky, e.g. recent publications concerning medication compliance.

(2) In specifying and selecting the study sample:
(a) *Popularity bias*. The admission of patients to some practices, institutions, or procedures (surgery, autopsy) is influenced by the interest stirred up by the presenting condition and its possible causes, e.g. White: *Brit Med J*. 2: 1284–1288, 1953.
(b) *Centripetal bias*. The reputations of certain clinicians and institutions cause individuals with specific disorders or exposure to gravitate toward them, e.g. the striking rate of posterior fossa cerebral aneurysms reported from the University of Western Ontario.
(c) *Referral filter bias*. As a group of ill are referred from primary to secondary to tertiary care, the concentration of rare causes, multiple diagnoses, and "hopeless cases" may increase, e.g. secondary

hypertension at the Cleveland Clinic; Gifford: *Milbank Mem Fund Quart* 47: 170–186, 1969.

(d) *Diagnostic access bias*. Individuals differ in their geographic, temporal, and economic access to the diagnostic procedures that label them as having a given disease, e.g. Andersen, Andersen: Patterns of use of health services. In: *Handbook of Medical Sociology*. Freeman et al. (Eds). Englewood Cliffs: Prentice-Hall, 1972.

(e) *Diagnostic suspicion bias*. A knowledge of the subject's prior exposure to a putative cause (ethnicity, taking a certain drug, having a second disorder, being exposed in an epidemic) may influence both the intensity and the outcome of the diagnostic process, e.g. the possibility that rubber workers were victims of this bias was studied by Fox, White: *Lancet* 1: 1009–1010, 1976.

(f) *Unmasking (detection signal) bias*. An innocent exposure may become suspect if, rather than causing a disease, it causes a sign or symptom which precipitates a search for the disease, e.g. the current controversy over post-menopausal estrogens and cancer of the endometrium.

(g) *Mimicry bias*. An innocent exposure may become suspect if, rather than causing a disease, it causes a (benign) disorder which resembles the disease, e.g. Morrison et al. *Lancet* 1: 1142–1143, 1977.

(h) *Previous opinion bias*. The tactics and results of a previous diagnostic process on a patient, e.g. multiple personal experiences with referred hypertensive patients.

(i) *Wrong sample size bias*. Samples which are too small can prove nothing; samples which are too large can prove anything.

(j) *Admission rate (Berkson) bias*. If hospitalization rates differ for different exposure/disease groups, the relation between exposure and disease will become distorted in hospital-based studies. Berkson: *Biometrics Bull* 2: 47–53, 1946; Roberts RS, Spitzer WO, Delmore T, Sackett DL: *J Chron Dis* 31: 119–128.

(k) *Prevalence–incidence (Neyman) bias*. A late look at those exposed (or affected) early will miss fatal and other short episodes, plus mild or "silent" cases and cases in which evidence of exposure disappears with disease onset. Neyman: *Science* 122: 401, 1955.

(l) *Diagnostic vogue bias*. The same illness may receive different diagnostic labels at different points in space or time, e.g. British "bronchitis" versus North American "emphysema": Fletcher et al.: *Amer Rev Resp Dis* 90: 1–13, 1964.

(m) *Diagnostic purity bias*. When "pure" diagnostic groups exclude co-morbidity they may become non-representative.

(n) *Procedure selection bias*. Certain clinical procedures may be preferentially offered to those who are poor risks, e.g. selection of patients for "medical" versus "surgical" therapy; Feinstein: *Clin Biostatics* 76, 1976.

(o) *Missing clinical data bias*. Missing clinical data may be missing because they are normal, negative, never measured, or measured but never recorded.

(p) *Non-contemporaneous control bias*. Secular changes in definitions, exposures, diagnoses, diseases, and treatments may render non-contemporaneous controls non-comparable, e.g. Feinstein: *Clin Biostatistics*: 89–104, 1977.

(q) *Starting time bias*. The failure to identify a common starting time for exposure or illness may lead to systematic misclassification, e.g. Feinstein: *Clin Biostatistics*: 89–104, 1977.

(r) *Unacceptable disease bias*. When disorders are socially unacceptable (V.D., suicide, insanity) they tend to be under-reported.

(s) *Migrator bias*. Migrants may differ systematically from those who stay home, e.g. Krueger, Moriyama: *Amer J Publ Hlth* 57: 496–503, 1967.

(t) *Membership bias*. Membership in a group (the employed, joggers, etc.) may imply a degree of health which differs systematically from that of the general population, e.g. exercise and recurrent myocardial infarction. Rechnitzer et al.: *Circulation* 45: 853–857, 1972 and *J Roy Coll Phys*: 29–30, 1978.

(u) *Non-respondent bias*. Non-respondents (or "late comers") from a specified sample may exhibit exposures of outcomes which differ from those of respondents (or "early comers"), e.g. cigarette smokers; Seltzer et al.: *Amer J Epid* 100: 453–547, 1974.

(v) *Volunteer bias*. Volunteers or "early comers" from a specified sample may exhibit exposures or outcomes (they tend to be healthier) which differ from those of non-volunteers or "late comers," e.g. volunteers for screening: Shapiro et al.: JAMA 215: 1777–1785, 1971.

(3) In executing the experimental manoeuvre (or exposure):

(a) *Contamination bias*. In an experiment when members of the control group inadvertently receive the experimental manoeuvre, the difference in outcomes between experimental and control patients may be systematically reduced, e.g. recent drug trials involving aspirin.

(b) *Withdrawal bias*. Patients who are withdrawn from an experiment may differ systematically from those who remain, e.g. in a neurosurgical trial of surgical versus medical therapy of cerebrovascular disease, patients who died or stroked-out during surgery were withdrawn as "unavailable for follow-up" and excluded from early analyses.

(c) *Compliance bias.* In experiments requiring patient adherence to therapy, issues of efficacy become confounded with those of compliance, e.g. it is the high risk coronary patients who quit exercise programs; Oldridge et al.: *Canad Med Assoc J* 118: 361–364, 1978.

(d) *Therapeutic personality bias.* When treatment is not "blind," the therapist's convictions about efficacy may systematically influence both outcomes (positive personality) and their measurement (desire for positive results).

(e) *Bogus control bias.* When patients who are allocated to an experimental manoeuvre die or sicken before or during its administration and are omitted or re-allocated to the control group, the experimental manoeuvre will appear spuriously superior.

(4) In measuring exposures and outcomes:

(a) *Intensive measure bias.* When outcome measures are incapable of detecting clinically significant changes or differences, Type II errors occur.

(b) *Underlying cause bias (rumination bias).* Cases may ruminate about possible causes for their illnesses and thus exhibit different recall or prior exposures than controls, e.g. Sartwell: Ann Int Med 81: 381–386, 1974 (see also the Recall bias).

(c) *End-digit preference bias.* In converting analog to digital data, observers may record some terminal digits with an unusual frequency, e.g. a notorious problem in the measurement of blood pressure; Rose et al.: *Lancet* 1:296–300, 1964.

(d) *Apprehension bias.* Certain measures (pulse, blood pressure) may alter systematically from their usual levels when the subject is apprehensive, e.g. blood pressure during medical interviews; McKegney, Williams: Amer J Psychiat 123: 1539–1545, 1967.

(e) *Unacceptability bias.* Measurements which hurt, embarrass, or invade privacy may be systematically refused or evaded.

(f) *Obsequiousness bias.* Subjects may systematically alter questionnaire responses in the direction they perceive desired by the investigator.

(g) *Expectation bias.* Observers may systematically err in measuring and recording observations so that they concur with prior expectations, e.g. house officers tend to report "normal" fetal heart rates; Day et al.: *Brit Med J* 4:422–424, 1968.

(h) *Substitution game.* The substitution of a risk factor which has not been established as causal for it associated outcome. Yerushalmy: In: *Controversy*

in Internal Medicine. Ingelfinger et al. (Eds). 1966.

(i) *Family information bias.* The flow of family information about exposure and illness is stimulated by, and directed to, a new case in its midst, e.g. different family histories of arthritis from affected an unaffected sib.; Schull, Cobb: J Chron Dis 22: 217–222, 1969.

(j) *Exposure suspicion bias.* A knowledge of the subject's disease status may influence both the intensity and outcome of a search for exposure to the putative cause, e.g. Sartwell: *Ann Int Med* 81: 381–386, 1974.

(k) *Recall bias.* Questions about specific exposures may be asked several times of cases but only once of controls. (See also the underlying cause bias.)

(l) *Attention bias.* Study subjects may systematically alter their behavior when they know they are being observed, e.g. Hawthorne revisited.

(m)*Instrument bias.* Defects in the calibration or maintenance of measurement instruments may lead to systematic deviations from true values.

(5) In analyzing the data:

(a) *Post-hoc significance bias.* When decision levels or "tails" for a and b are selected *after* the data have been examined, conclusions may be biased.

(b) Data dredging bias (looking for the pony). When data are reviewed for all possible associations without prior hypothesis, the results are suitable for hyposthesis-forming activities only.

(c) *Scale degradation bias.* The degradation and collapsing of measurement instruments may lead to systematic deviations from true values.

(d) *Tidying-up bias.* The exclusion of outlyers or other untidy results cannot be justified on statistical grounds and may lead to bias, e.g. Murphy: *The Logic of Medicine*: p. 250, 1976.

(e) *Repeated peeks bias.* Repeated peeks at accumulating data in a randomized trial are not dependent and may lead to inappropriate termination.

(6) In interpreting the analysis:

(a) *Mistaken identity bias.* In compliance trials, strategies directed toward improving the patient's compliance may, instead or in addition, cause the treating clinician to prescribe more vigorously: the effect upon achievement of the treatment goal may be misinterpreted, e.g. Sackett: Priorities and methods for future research. In: Compliance with Therapeutic Regimens. Sackett DL, Haynes RB (Eds). 1976.

(b) *Cognitive dissonance bias.* The belief in a given mechanism may increase rather than decrease in the face of contradictory evidence, e.g. Sackett: How can we improve patient compliance? In:

Controversies in Therapeutics. Lasagna L (Ed). In press.

(c) *Magnitude bias.* In interpreting a finding the selection of a scale of measurement may markedly affect the interpretation, e.g. $1,000,000 may also be 0.0003% of the national budget; Murphy: *The Logic of Medicine*: p. 249, 1976.

(d) *Significance bias.* The confusion of statistical significance, on the one hand, with biologic or clinical or health care significance, on the other hand, can lead to fruitless studies and useless conclusions, e.g. Feinstein: *Clin Biostatistics*, p. 258, 1977.

(e) *Correlation bias.* Equating correlation with causation leads to errors of both kinds, e.g. Hill: *Principles of Medical Statistics.* 9th ed. pp. 309–320, 1971.

(f) Under-exhaustion bias. The failure to exhaust the hypothesis space may lead to authoritarian rather than authoritative interpretation, e.g. Murphy: *The Logic of Medicine*: p. 258, 1976.

Index

SUNY HEALTH SCIENCES LIB. - SYRACUSE

3 2803 00255827 7

WB 25 B328c 2001
Batavia, Mitch/Clinical
research for health

M

X